What's My Age Again?

The science of skin, ageing, and confidence–decoded

Jemma Hicks

Published by Vivid Publishing
A division of Fontaine Publishing Group
P.O. Box 948, Fremantle
Western Australia 6959
www.vividpublishing.com.au

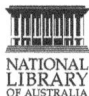

A catalogue record for this
book is available from the
National Library of Australia

Contents

I want to dedicate this book to my dad, Darren Gleeson, and my husband, Joshua Hicks.

Dad - You inspire me every day to dream bigger than I ever could have imagined. A successful multiple business owner and franchisor with over 100 franchisees, a published author, a man who has climbed Everest nearly annually for the last few years just for fun, and most importantly, a dedicated Dad.

Josh - My husband and supporter. Thank you for putting up with my constant crazy ideas and work ethic, which can be overwhelming at times, as I'm always busy. Thank you for holding everything down for me while I'm in a whirlwind.

Without both of you, this wouldn't have been possible.

Hi, I'm Jemma. A registered nurse, cosmetic injector, wife, friend, and confessed skin obsessive who's always deep diving into the latest trends, treatments, and ingredients.

My journey started right after high school in Bunbury, WA. At 17, I had no idea where life would take me. I chose ATAR subjects like psychology and biology simply because they sounded interesting, but I still wasn't sure what I wanted to do. A friend mentioned nursing, a career that could take me anywhere in the world and the thought of working in places like London or Paris had me hooked. Without ever having stepped foot in a hospital, I signed up for a three-year nursing degree and threw myself into it completely.

At the time, I was convinced I'd become a midwife. I even applied for a graduate position at a children's and mothers' hospital, but when I didn't get the offer, I was crushed. Soon after, I completed a six-week rural placement that rotated through surgical, maternity, emergency, and theatre, and I had a huge realisation: midwifery wasn't for me after all. I found myself drawn instead to surgical and emergency nursing, and it felt like everything was falling into place.

I started my nursing career bright-eyed and bushy-tailed at just 20 years old, working my graduate year in medical and stroke rehab. Sadly, right before starting my second rotation, my Pa suffered a stroke. Treating other patients while wanting to be by his side was one of the hardest challenges of my career, but it gave me a deeper perspective and a lot of resilience.

Soon after, I moved to a tertiary hospital for more experience on a busy surgical and vascular ward. It was fast-paced, intense, and rewarding, but my lifelong eczema started catching up with me. After months of cracked, weeping hands from constant washing, gloves, and sanitiser, I spent a year trialling ointments, wraps, and even diet changes. Eventually, my dermatologist told me, *"You're allergic to the hospital. You need to find a new career."* I was devastated.

After some soul-searching (and plenty of late-night Googling), I discovered cosmetic nursing, a field I had never considered before but instantly intrigued me. I enrolled in a postgraduate diploma, took on a trainee injector role, and continued working hospital shifts while studying part-time. Life was chaotic, with workdays stretching up to six days a week, often juggling hospital, clinic, and coursework responsibilities all in one day. Still, I knew I was investing in my future, and that kept me going.

Fast forward to today: I've now been a cosmetic nurse for eight years, working in some of Perth's most respected injectable clinics before opening my own. My business has now grown to two clinics, Karrinyup and Ellenbrook, and trades as *Skin Societé*. Alongside my business partner, who owns other clinics across WA, we focus on education, innovation, and helping clients understand the "why" behind their skin changes. We believe great results come from a holistic approach combining tailored in-clinic treatments, at-home skincare, advanced laser therapies, and, where appropriate, targeted supplements to support skin health from the inside out.

This is more than a career for me, it's my passion. My goal is to empower clients with knowledge so they can make informed decisions and feel confident in their own skin.

1

Introduction to Skin & Aging

A common thing I hear from my clients when they come in is "one day I woke up and I look old" or "this line only just appeared". It may seem like the line appeared in your sleep while you are running through your chaotic life. Whether that be surviving motherhood, trying to beat that deadline for work or getting caught up in the day-to-day. But it's caused by a cascade of small changes that start to happen in our mid-twenties (Yes, twenties?!). These changes eventually cause our skin to begin to sag and gain a few extra lines than we previously had.

So, what is happening?

SKIN ANATOMY

As you probably already know, our skin is one of the largest organs in our body. So, of course, we must take great care of it. Our skin has many functions, such as providing our organs with a protective barrier from chemicals, physical and mechanical harm. Another role of skin is to control and regulate our body temperature. Our body is very adaptive and excellent at adjusting to accommodate external fluctuations. Blood vessels can be dilated (expand) to cool us down or constricted (tighten up) to heat us. The skin also allows us to absorb essential vitamins, such as facilitating the synthesis of vitamin D from the sun and absorbing our skincare to boost hydration. And lastly, it is also an effective method of waste disposal for the body in the form of sweat. Sweating is an effective way to cool the body down by releasing liquid from our sweat glands. When the wind blows upon our skin, it assists with temperature regulation by cooling us down. Sweat can also contain nitrogenous waste and salt (unwanted molecules), so they don't build up in our bodies.

As you age, you will notice that your skin becomes thinner and develops a more wrinkled appearance. Our skin is comprised of many different layers of different types of skin cells. We often talk about the top layer, which is the stratum corneum, as this is the outermost layer of the skin and makes up what we see. This is comprised of fifteen to thirty layers of skin cells, stacked on top of each other, interwoven and compressed. So, when we are talking about chemical peeling (taking off a layer or two of skin cells), don't worry, as it's really such a small amount of what we have. The stratum corneum has many functions, such as waterproofing the skin, ensuring that water cannot get in or out of the body (unless via specialised sweat glands). Maintaining the health of our stratum corneum is vital to having a healthy skin barrier and protecting our internals from trauma such as abrasions and wounds. We will discuss what an impaired skin barrier is and the impact it has on you in a later chapter.

Deeper down in the skin, we have the dermis. This is comprised of firm but flexible connective tissue, a healthy blood supply and accessory structures. Clinic treatments (such as dermal therapies) can activate processes in the dermis by stimulating fibroblasts within this layer. Fibroblasts play a key role in wound healing, providing structural support and elasticity. The dermis contains collagen and elastin fibres that provide structure to the skin. These are often buzzwords that we hear and see on products that draw us in to buy them. But why are they important? Collagen is a protein present in most connective tissues and is produced by fibroblasts. Fibroblasts also make elastic fibres and provide resistance to the skin, allowing it to stretch and recoil.

From the age of twenty-five years, our collagen, elastin, and fibroblasts begin to decrease around 1% to 1.5% per year (Reilly and Lozano, 2021). You can imagine how this small percentage can really start to accumulate annually. And this can, of course, be accelerated by various external factors such as smoking, UV sun exposure, diet, and hydration.

Many factors can also affect our collagen and elastin levels over time. It is not all due to age; it can also be affected by UV sun exposure, chemicals and stress levels. And of course, intrinsic factors such as our genetic predisposition and ethnicity. That is why we often follow a similar pattern of ageing as our relatives, despite varying extrinsic factors.

Collagen fibres become damaged over time as they are utilised within the body. This, of course, restricts the effectiveness of the bounce, recoil, and structure that they create for the skin. As we age, the skin will begin to atrophy (become thinner), and the quantity and quality of our collagen, elastin, and fibroblasts can decrease. The skin loses its firmness and becomes thinner, leading to a cumulative sagging effect (Reilly and Lozano, 2021). Hyaluronic acid levels within our skin also begin decreasing at a similar time. Hyaluronic acid (also known as HA) is a molecule present in our skin that retains hydration (H_2O). HA can hold multiple times its own weight in water, which can keep our skin feeling hydrated, dewy and youthful. If we lack sufficient water in our skin, which is naturally thinning, it's clear how this can lead to an impaired barrier.

Oxidative stress is one of the most significant drivers of skin aging. It is caused by an imbalance between free radicals and the body's ability to neutralise them with readily available antioxidants. Free radicals are unstable molecules generated by everyday factors like UV exposure, pollution, smoking, poor nutrition, and even stress. Over time, these molecules damage skin cells, proteins, and lipids, accelerating the breakdown of collagen and elastin while impairing the skin's natural repair mechanisms. This can lead to visible signs of aging, including fine lines, dullness, pigmentation, and sagging tissues.

Supporting your skin's natural antioxidant defences is an integral part of maintaining long-term skin health. A balanced diet rich in antioxidants, such as vitamins A, C, and E, combined with targeted skincare products containing antioxidant-rich ingredients, can help to reduce free radical damage in the skin. This means eating a diverse, nutrient-rich diet, focusing on increasing your intake of vegetables, fruits, nuts and lean proteins. Protecting the skin from excessive sun exposure with daily SPF is also one of the most effective ways to reduce oxidative stress and maintain healthy, youthful-looking skin over time.

BONE REABSORPTION

As we age, one of the most significant yet often overlooked changes occurs deep beneath the skin—in the skeletal structure of the face. The zygomatic bone, commonly known as the cheekbone, plays a key role in the mid-face's structure and appearance. It provides vital support for the overlying soft tissues and determines the natural projection of the eyes, cheeks, and surrounding features. Over time, bones can undergo resorption, a process where the body gradually breaks down and reabsorbs bone tissue. This can result in a loss of volume and structural support in critical areas of the facial skeleton, particularly around the eye sockets, cheeks, and jawline. These subtle shifts affect not only the face's contour but also the positioning of fat pads and muscles, which can contribute to a more hollowed, aged appearance.

Bone resorption impacts the anchoring of the superficial musculoaponeurotic system (SMAS), a fibrous network that connects facial muscles to the skin. As the underlying bone diminishes, soft tissue begins to sag and descend, which can make the skin appear lax and less supported. These changes can lead to deeper nasolabial folds (the lines from the nose to the corners of the mouth), sunken eyes, reduced projection in the mid-face, and often jowls along the jawline. While these changes are part of the natural aging process, understanding the role of the facial skeleton helps explain why simply tightening the skin is often not enough to give you the results you at looking for. Modern aesthetic treatments now aim to restore lost volume and rebuild structural support, rather than focusing solely on surface correction. There has been growing popularity with improving skin health over recent years, as a deeper understanding and more education are available around the anatomical changes of ageing and appropriate prevention measures.

SUBCUTANEOUS TISSUE

Another major contributor to the visual signs of facial aging is the change in structure and rearrangement of fat pads. In youth, facial fat is evenly distributed in well-defined compartments that create a naturally lifted and smooth contour. However, with age, these fat pads can lose volume and begin to descend, contributing to sagging, hollowness, and the deepening of facial folds. This change in fat distribution inverts the so-called **"triangle of youth"**, where youthful features—full cheeks and a narrow jawline—are replaced by flat cheeks, jowls, and heaviness in the lower face.

Facial fat is not a single mass but is divided into distinct anatomical compartments, both deep and superficial. These compartments do not age uniformly; some areas lose volume more quickly than others, which can result in uneven contours, under-eye hollowing, and mid-face deflation. This compartmentalised aging is why certain areas, like the tear trough or cheeks, may appear more sunken or tired, even if other parts of the face remain relatively unchanged. Additionally, because these fat pads act as cushions and supportive layers, their shift or shrinkage directly affects how the skin drapes over the face. Understanding the specific anatomy of fat compartments helps practitioners address aging in a targeted, natural-looking way—by replenishing volume strategically, rather than overfilling or chasing wrinkles. Aesthetic treatments are often used to support these key fat compartments, which can help restore youthful proportions and balance to the face.

HORMONAL CHANGES

Hormones can fluctuate many times throughout our lives (even more so for women) and can cause many changes to occur in our skin. In our teenage years, a rapid increase in progesterone and testosterone increases oil production, which in turn can lead to oily skin and blocked pores. When the increased oil mixes with bacteria on the skin and dead skin cells, this causes inflammation and acne. Acne and inflammation often trigger each other, making both worse, which can feel like a never-ending loop. But with the right treatments and skincare, it can be tackled and appropriately controlled.

As we enter adulthood, these hormones begin to plateau, leading to a decrease in oil production. Some women may experience recurring periods of breakouts on their skin in accordance with their hormonal cycle around the time of their period. This is especially prevalent in women who suffer from PCOS. Polycystic Ovary Syndrome, also known as PCOS, is a condition of excess androgens (male hormones) that can lead to multiple cysts in the ovaries, inflammation, irregularity of periods, weight gain and acne (Chandravathi et al., 2015).

As we reach midlife and experience the decline of our hormones and menopause, we notice changes in our skin, too. As our hormones begin to decrease, we see our skin becoming drier and thinner, and our nails more brittle. We have a decrease in Estrogen and progesterone, paired with an increase in cortisol and inflammation, which can leave us feeling flat, dull and dry.

Throughout life, we experience many different changes due to the rise and fall of our hormones. This can affect how we look and feel about ourselves. With the right advice, treatment, and care, we can adjust throughout these periods to adapt to changes that make the process more manageable and comfortable.

2

Impaired Skin Barrier: Eczema, Psoriasis

Our skin is the largest organ in our body, and a very important one at that. It separates what is outside from what is contained inside and makes every attempt to keep it that way. Our skin reduces impact to protect our organs, prevents chemical exposure that may result in harm and keeps all of our body fluids inside where they should be. But due to various factors such as environmental stressors, pathogens, allergens and water loss, this vital barrier can become impaired.

WHAT MAKES UP THE SKIN BARRIER?

Many layers make up our skin. At the very top, we have our epidermis. This is the outermost layer, which is what we see. This is comprised of many compacted skin cells but is only around 0.8-1.4mm thick. The thickness of this layer varies all over the body. The soles of your feet and palms of your hands are the thickest layers in the body, and the skin around the eyes is one of the thinnest. This is due to the function of the skin in these areas. Keratin is produced in this layer by keratinocyte cells. Keratin plays an essential role in adding more structure to the skin, but this layer is also flexible and can absorb up to three times its own weight in water. However, if this layer dries out (water content falls below 10%), the skin's pliability reduces. This is why it is so important to keep the skin hydrated to reduce the appearance of fine lines and increase the skin's elasticity. The cells within the epidermal layer are held together via a viscous lipid layer that also assists with hydrating the skin.

The epidermis (outermost layer) contains multiple cells that work together to protect the skin and keep it functioning. Keratinocytes are in this layer and produce the fibrous protein keratin that gives our skin more structure. Melanocytes produce melanin, a brown pigment in our skin. This can determine our skin colour and is responsible for creating darker patches of skin (pigmentation). This will be discussed in more detail in a later chapter. Marker cells function as our touch receptors in association with our sensory nerve endings. They allow us to touch and feel our surroundings. And lastly, Langerhans cells, these are our macrophages (they are the exterminators: removing and destroying debris and bacteria) that help to activate our immune system. Essentially, this means that if something gets into the epidermal layer, such as debris from an injury or microorganism, it works like a garbage truck to encapsulate and remove it to maintain homeostasis.

In the upper layers of your skin, lamellar bodies are created inside skin cells. These tiny "packages" are filled with helpful fats, enzymes, and protective proteins. They help your skin stay strong and healthy. When your skin gets a signal like a rise in calcium, these lamellar bodies move to the edge of the skin cell and release their contents into the spaces between cells. This process helps form the skin barrier that protects you from the outside world. Once released, the fats inside are changed into ceramides, fatty acids, and cholesterol — three essential ingredients that keep your skin soft, hydrated, and firm. These fats then line up in neat layers between the skin cells, like bricks and mortar, to lock in moisture and keep out germs and irritants. This barrier is a big reason your skin can protect you, stay hydrated, and repair itself when damaged. The skin controls the release of water from the skin via the process of trans epidermal water loss or TEWL (Proksch, Brandner and Jensen, 2008).

SIGNS OF A DAMAGED SKIN BARRIER

An impaired skin barrier is often described as a high rate of trans epidermal water loss (TEWL) in the stratum corneum at a rate that cannot be replenished. This causes the skin to become dry, impacting its integrity and potentially leading to micro-openings or tears. This creates a direct passage for chemicals, pathogens, and debris to enter the skin and disrupt homeostasis.

This can be identified in the skin with the following symptoms.

- Increased sensitivity or stinging
- Dryness, flaking, tightness
- Redness and inflammation
- Increased breakouts or rashes
- Delayed healing

In some inherited conditions, the skin barrier is mildly impaired due to missing or faulty proteins like filaggrin, which helps form a strong and resilient skin surface. These people often have dry, flaky skin even without inflammation.

In more severe inflammatory skin conditions, such as eczema, psoriasis, and dermatitis, the barrier damage is more pronounced. These diseases show signs like dryness, scaling, itchiness and increased water loss through the skin (called TEWL – trans epidermal water loss).

CAUSES OF SKIN BARRIER IMPAIRMENT

As stated above, various factors affect our skin's ability to protect us. Main reasons for this include:

The overuse of active ingredients: This includes skincare products such as vitamin A (Retinol) and acids (think Glycolic and Salicylic). When introducing strong skincare products like these, it's crucial to start at a low percentage, just a day or two per week, and gradually increase as your skin tolerates. If too high a strength is used too frequently, it can disrupt the skin barrier, leading to dry, irritated, red skin, and in some cases, even increase breakouts.

Harsh cleansers or exfoliation: We need to ensure we are using a cleanser that is appropriate for our skin type to cleanse our skin thoroughly, but not in a way that's too harsh and potentially strips the skin of hydration. If your skin feels instantly tight and itchy after getting out of the shower, it's likely because your cleanser is too harsh or you have an impaired barrier. If you have sensitive skin or are experiencing this issue, I recommend avoiding gel cleansers (which are usually more stripping), products with acids, and anything containing exfoliating granules or microbeads. These can create micro tears in the skin, allowing pathogens and dirt to enter and water to escape. A cream, balm or oil cleanser can be soothing and more hydrating for irritated skin.

Environmental stress: Wintertime can cause our skin to become impaired due to the considerable variation in temperatures that we are exposed to. For example, when you try to warm your body up on a cold day by having a steaming hot shower. This significant variation in temperature from cold to hot can stress the skin, and the hot shower can increase the rate of TEWL, therefore leaving the skin dehydrated and irritated if not immediately nourished with moisturiser. Additionally, spending extended periods indoors with the air conditioner or heater on, which expels dry air, can quickly dry out your skin and make you feel more dehydrated. Adding moisture to the air with a humidifier can assist with this.

Stress: High cortisol levels produced by stress trigger a worsening of chronic diseases such as eczema and psoriasis. Studies have also found that higher levels of stress are linked to an increased rate of itching and itching sensation, which results in an increased rate of tissue damage and, therefore, barrier disruption (Evers and Beugen, 2021).

When we experience psychological or environmental stress, our brain and body respond in powerful ways that affect the skin. The connection between the brain and skin is often referred to as the "brain-skin axis." Here's how it works:

THE STRESS RESPONSE PATHWAY

1. Mental stress triggers a response in the brain's hypothalamic-pituitary-adrenal (HPA) axis.
2. This leads to the release of hormones like corticotropin-releasing hormone (CRH), ACTH, and prolactin (PRL).

3. These hormones can increase the release of stress-related chemicals such as substance P and calcitonin gene-related peptide (CGRP) from nerve endings.
4. These signals reach the skin, where the local production of CRH, ACTH, and glucocorticoids (stress hormones) increases.
5. This can cause inflammation, skin sensitivity, and flare-ups of skin conditions.

THE ROLE OF MAST CELLS AND NERVE FIBRES

In the skin, mast cells act as key "switches" in this stress response. They are sensitive to stress signals and can release substances that cause inflammation and itchiness. Stress also encourages the growth of new nerve fibres in the skin, which can heighten sensitivity (Arck et al., 2006).

THE BODY'S IMMUNE SHIFT

Stress hormones like glucocorticoids change how your immune system behaves. They can:

- Suppress specific immune responses that fight infection (called Th1 responses),
- While increasing others that are associated with allergies and inflammation (called Th2 responses).

This shift can protect the body from excessive inflammation but may also make it more susceptible to allergic or inflammatory skin conditions like eczema and psoriasis.

OTHER KEY STRESS PLAYERS:

- Prolactin supports immune cell survival during stress.
- The sympathetic nervous system, which releases adrenaline and noradrenaline, also affects immune cells by altering their movement and activity.
- Nerve Growth Factor (NGF), another critical molecule, helps nerve growth and increases inflammation in the skin by encouraging immune cell activity.

Chronic stress doesn't just impact your mood; it literally changes how your skin behaves and can weaken the skin barrier, increase inflammation, and trigger or worsen skin conditions. This is why managing stress is just as crucial for healthy skin as using good skincare products.

Hormones: The decrease in estrogen levels during menopause negatively impacts the skin's water-holding abilities by decreasing the amount of hyaluronic acid we have. This also reduces our production of collagen and elastin. This makes our skin more dehydrated and fragile, making it susceptible to damage and dullness.

MEDICAL CONDITIONS RELATED TO BARRIER DYSFUNCTION

➤ Eczema (Atopic Dermatitis)

Eczema is one of the most common skin conditions seen by dermatologists. It causes itchy, inflamed, and often dry skin. Various genetic as well as environmental factors can contribute to a flare-up of eczema.

Genetic: Pathological changes may include: *spongiosis* - an overproduction of hyaluronic acid, release of galectin-7, and reduced E-cadherin. Spongiosis is when there is an excess of hyaluronic acid in the epidermis, resulting in oedema (too much fluid) in this layer. This condition is characterised by the formation of small pustules on the surface of the skin. Galectin-7 contributes to processes that result in cell death, cell migration and cell adhesion. All of which are essential processes in the cell life cycle and crucial for healthy skin.

Environmental: There are many different things in your environment that can add to an eczema flare. Common causes include rapid temperature fluctuations, increased dry air, friction, and fragrances and essential oils found in skincare, makeup, and cleaning products. Other causes may be simply due to sweating. This warm, moist environment can result in the breakdown of skin in areas such as the inner elbows and behind the knees. But a flare-up can also be caused by cool, dry temperatures in which the skin becomes dry and may crack due to dehydration in winter, allowing irritants to enter and disrupt the balance.

TEWL (transepidermal water loss) is increased in people suffering from eczema as a factor that contributes to the dehydration of the skin. Corticosteroids are a commonly prescribed medication for eczema that are known to be effective. However, it's essential to understand that this medication can only be used short-term, as long-term use can cause increasing issues such as Topical steroid withdrawal (TSW). Topical treatment with corticosteroids is shown to reduce the water loss in clients with eczema due to a decrease in dilation of blood vessels in the area, which would be a usual response to an irritant. It decreases the usual inflammatory tissue response, which in turn reduces redness, swelling, oozing and flaking.

In eczema, many people have a genetic issue with their skin barrier even before visible rashes appear. Mutations in the filaggrin gene are a strong risk factor — about 1 in 5 people with eczema have this mutation, and it's even more common in severe cases. This allows allergens and irritants to penetrate the skin more easily, which triggers inflammation.

➤ **Psoriasis**

Psoriasis is a genetic, lifelong inflammatory disease characterised by plaque, flexural, guttate, pustular, or erythrodermic psoriasis. It causes thick plaques, redness and flaking of the skin that can be both embarrassing and debilitating for the client.

Types of psoriasis include:
- Plaque: Itchy, dry, covered with scales
- Flexural: Localised to skin folds and genitals
- Guttate: Small scaling spots on the trunk and limbs. Common in children post-streptococcus infection.
- Pustular: Blisters with pus
- Erythrodermic: Red rash over most of the body

(Dhabale and Nagpure, 2022)

Psoriasis is an autoimmune condition, so flare-ups are possible at any time. The client needs to reduce known triggers. Flare-ups result in an overproduction of skin cells, which impairs the skin cycle and leads to hardened, discoloured plaques on the skin in clusters. Common triggers can include stress, infection and injury. The skin's outermost layer lacks essential lipids such as ceramides that can impede its function, which in turn increases the rate of TEWL and dries the skin out (Raharja, Mahil and Barker, 2021).

► **Rosacea**

Rosacea is a common chronic skin condition that's exhibited by erythema, papules, pustules, telangiectasias, flushing, phymatous changes, and ocular manifestations.

There is no current cure for rosacea, so management and treatment regimens are designed to suppress the inflammatory lesions, erythema, and, to a lesser extent, the telangiectasia involved with rosacea (Gupta and Chaudhry, 2005). Common triggers for Rosacea include sudden temperature changes, spicy food, alcohol, and certain skincare ingredients, such as astringents (moisture-stripping ingredients). IPL and laser treatments can be effective in treating the broken capillaries on the surface of the skin. Mild and calming skincare is beneficial in decreasing redness and inflammation to soothe the skin. If the condition remains uncontrolled despite these attempts, you may require treatment from your GP.

THE ROLE OF THE MICROBIOME

The skin has a microbiome, like the one in our gut. Many different types of microbes inhabit the skin to keep it happy and balanced. Skin flora plays an essential role in defending the skin barrier from outside pathogens. Factors contributing to variation in the skin microbiota include the density of hair follicles and glands (sweat or sebaceous), host factors (such as age and sex) and environmental factors (such as occupation, climate and hygiene) (Grice and Segre, 2011). The skin microbiome works by warding off external pathogens and alerting the immune system when it becomes under threat.

Some microbes can even make the skin more acidic to prevent bacterial growth. Prebiotics and probiotics are essential for a happy skin microbiome. Probiotics are live microorganisms, such as bacteria, that reside on the skin to maintain its balance. Prebiotics serve as food for these probiotics. Dybiosis is a shift or change in the microbiome that can cause it to become unbalanced, which can result in a flare-up of skin conditions. This can be a result of chemical exposure, environmental factors, diet, infection, and antibiotics. When the skin is impaired, introducing skincare with prebiotics and probiotics can be beneficial. This improves the skin microbiome, assisting with wound healing and reducing the frequency and severity of breakouts. Additionally, it enhances barrier quality and minimises sensitivity.

IMPACT OF AESTHETIC TREATMENTS

When you come in for your skin consultation, the nurse or dermal therapist will do a thorough skin analysis and, in some instances, complete a photographed assessment using tools such as the Observ machine or wood's lamp. They are assessing skin quality, pigmentation, signs of age and breakouts, but most importantly, they are observing the health of your skin. They will evaluate for any redness, irritation, breaks in the skin, or signs of infection before any dermal therapies, such as peels, lasers, and micro needling. If signs of skin breakdown, such as those listed above, are present, it is not considered safe or smart to proceed with any dermal therapies on that day. Depending on the flare-up, it may be suitable to either postpone the treatment or change it to a facial with calming steps, such as hydrating serums, probiotic masks, and LED light therapy, to help reduce and calm inflammation. It is not advised to use water that is too hot during this time, apply any acids for exfoliation to the skin or use highly scented products, as they may all contribute to worsening an impaired barrier.

For clients with chronic eczema that never seems to go away (i.e. settling for only short periods of time), I recommend testing a small 1cm section of skin with the desired product for its anti-aging benefits. It's crucial to leave the product on the skin for a minute or two (if suitable, leave on – depending on the product) and wait until the next day before assessing whether the skin will respond positively or negatively to that product. I would always recommend applying the test patch to the skin between the ear and the jawline. This way, if the client reacts to the product, it will be less noticeable and cause less friction to the area, resulting in quicker healing.

SUPPORTING AND REPAIRING THE SKIN BARRIER

Gentle fragrance-free cream cleansers are recommended as they are often the least irritating and most hydrating for the skin. You can even find some with added beneficial ingredients such as hyaluronic acid and ceramides.

Barrier-supporting ingredients:
- o **Ceramides:** Natural oils found in the skin (making up to 50% of the oils) that assist with reducing dehydration in the skin.
- o **Niacinamide:** Also known as vitamin B. It hydrates the skin while also decreasing excessive oil production. It improves the barrier function of the skin.
- o **Fatty acids:** Hydrate and maintain skin barrier
- o **Hyaluronic acid:** Water-holding properties to help hydrate the skin.
- o **Zinc:** Helps to soothe and calm. Strengthens the skin.

It is essential to choose the correct type of moisturiser for your skin's requirements. Whether you're breakout-prone or tend to be on the drier side. There is always a moisturiser to keep you glowing.

Common moisturiser types:

Humectant moisturisers often contain glycerine and work by attracting moisture from the air around them. This can help bring more water into the skin to increase hydration. They are usually lightweight and very comfortable to wear.

Occlusive moisturisers are very thick and create a barrier or shield between the skin and the outside environment. If you are dry before application, it can be beneficial to apply a hydrating serum so the occlusive moisturiser can lock that hydration in. These moisturisers have a thick texture, making them unsuitable for clients with acne, as they may cause discomfort until fully absorbed.

Topical steroids are a commonly prescribed medication when it comes to eczema and dermatitis. They work by decreasing inflammation in the skin and can decrease proliferation (new cell growth), which can be effective for skin that is over proliferating. However, overuse can lead to withdrawal effects and skin thinning. It is recommended to treat eczema and dermatitis with skincare first, before commencing corticosteroids. Start with the smallest percentage and ideally apply it over a moisturiser to further dilute it.

LIFESTYLE FACTORS

There are several actions the client can take to support their journey in preventing and minimising an impaired barrier. Eating a healthy diet and reducing processed foods can help reduce inflammation in the body. Inflammatory foods include dairy, gluten, sugar and highly processed foods. Aim to eat more fresh fruits, vegetables and healthy omega-3s. As always, it's recommended to drink two litres of water per day to hydrate you inside and out. You'd be surprised by how much water your skin holds. Increasing your water intake, if it is below the recommended amount, will significantly improve your skin's glow and hydration.

As discussed earlier in the chapter, stress plays a strong role in the inflammatory response in the skin, which could contribute to a breakdown in the barrier.

I always recommend to my clients that they reduce irritant contact with their skin and make every effort to minimise outbreaks. This can be achieved by using mild soap-free cleansers, gentle washing detergents, and cleaning products, and by choosing hypoallergenic products where possible. You'd be surprised by the number of products in your home that can be contributing to skin issues. When having a flare-up, it is important to have short showers and avoid extreme temperature changes, which can promote TEWL. We often recommend limiting showering to once per day during a flare and opting for a lukewarm shower when possible. When the barrier is impaired, your skin will likely feel parched as soon as you exit the shower. It is important to apply moisturisers and emollients within 3 minutes of leaving the shower to reduce the rate of TEWL and lock that hydration straight in.

Hot tip: I always recommend that my clients dry themselves to about ¾, leaving just a small amount of residual water on them. Then apply an ultra-hydrating but lightweight fragrance-free moisturiser all over to lock that hydration straight in. It may be beneficial to reapply moisturiser as required throughout the day.

PROFESSIONAL SKIN TREATMENTS THAT SUPPORT THE BARRIER

In clinic treatments that can be used to support the barrier function can include:

- **Barrier repair facials:** Fragrance-free calming facials that don't include any acids for exfoliation. Its focus is to nourish the skin and increase hydration.
- **LED light therapy:** A light-emitting device that focuses on encouraging wound healing, stimulating collagen and elastin production and, in the case of a blue light, killing bacteria on the skin. There are varying lights that can be chosen on the LED for different benefits:
  - **Red:** Stimulating collagen and elastin production.
  - **Yellow:** Promotes wound healing and decreases bruising.
  - **Blue:** Kills bacteria on the skin that contribute to acne.
  - **Green:** Assists with reducing pigmentation
- Enzyme masks: These masks are effective in increasing blood flow to the area, which can, in turn, improve wound healing.

PRESCRIPTION OR COSMECEUTICAL ROUTINES:

<u>Cleanser:</u> I recommend opting for a cream cleanser over a gel cleanser as it tends to be more hydrating and reduces the likelihood of that dry, tight feeling when you come out of the shower.

<u>Balancer:</u> A lightweight probiotic serum can be the perfect addition, as it can assist in balancing the microbiome on your skin. I like to tell my clients it's like a yakult for your face.

<u>Serum:</u> A hydrating fragrance-free serum, such as a hyaluronic acid, is beneficial in holding water in the skin.

<u>Hydrating fragrance-free moisturiser:</u> Look for a product with ceramides and an occlusive agent to keep your skin hydrated.

<u>SPF:</u> A crucial step for all. Many clients experience a stinging sensation from some chemical sunscreens that can cause inflammation, leading to redness and a burning sensation. I recommend opting for a physical zinc sunscreen instead, as I have found that I do not experience irritation from this type.

<u>Hydrating mask:</u> During periods of skin impairment and flare-ups, it can be beneficial to have weekly or twice-weekly hydrating probiotic masks to give that boost of hydration

and cool the skin.

Clients can also benefit from taking supplements such as fish oil, zinc and probiotics.

Fish oil: Omega-3s and essential fatty acids that hydrate the skin and maintain a healthy lipid balance.

Zinc: essential in maintaining the skin barrier

Probiotics: Happy gut - happy skin. Assists with maintaining a happy gut microbiome.

CLIENT EDUCATION AND HOME CARE

It is essential that once a client or clinician notices signs of barrier impairment, a calm and hydrating skin care routine is implemented to help get the skin back on track as soon as possible.

Top tips to get back to healthy skin:
- Avoid extreme changes in temperature.
- Apply moisturiser within 3 mins of getting out of the shower to lock in results.
- Drop back to a simple skincare routine when you experience irritation. Think cream cleanser, balancer, hydrating serum, moisturiser and SPF.
- Avoid active ingredients while your skin is irritated, as these exfoliate the skin and can exacerbate it.

- Avoid dairy, sugar and preservatives where possible.

Maintain consistency with a simplified routine, and over time, it will heal. You can't speed up the process, but you can provide a healing environment, and your skin will follow.

3

Acne: Not just the overproduction of oil

WHAT IS ACNE?

Acne is a chronic inflammatory condition of the skin, often arising during puberty, but it can also occur throughout various other times during a person's life. This condition is characterised by increased sebaceous activity (increased oil production), hyperkeratinisation (increased keratin production on the skin) and overproduction of P. acnes bacteria (Dréno, 2017). Numerous factors contribute to and exacerbate acne. Factors such as stress, over-exfoliation, increased sebaceous activity, certain cosmetic products, and dietary choices can all influence the skin's health.

As discussed, dysbiosis is a shift or change in the microbiome of your skin. This can result in an impaired skin barrier but can also contribute to the manifestation of acne on the skin. So how does this occur? As we know, the skin barrier can be disturbed by a variety of factors such as incorrect use or dosage of skincare products, over-exfoliation, chemical, environmental or hormonal influences. This results in the skin being out of balance and unable to effectively defend itself from external stressors. P. acnes bacteria, also known as Propionibacterium acnes, are a type of gram-positive bacterium that causes acne on the skin. The quantity of this bacterium proliferates during an outbreak of acne and triggers the inflammation cascade.

This condition is most prevalent during the years of puberty due to the massive surge in hormones that teenagers experience. Sex hormones are converted in the skin, stimulating the production of sebaceous glands and enhancing their size to allow for a larger flow of sebum.

It can also arise late in a person's life, typically in the mid to late twenties or thirties, during pregnancy, and at other times. These times often correlate with a surge in hormones, such as pregnancy, when the body is under a large amount of stress and hormones are changing, or from trialling a new type of hormonal contraception that may not agree with your body and therefore throw out the balance. And in some cases, which can be shocking to the client, can arise during the premenopausal stage of life, which is also heavily caused by a change in hormones, most commonly, the androgenous type (testosterone).

HOW ACNE DEVELOPS (THE ACNE CASCADE)

Many small changes in the body can lead to acne.

These changes include:
- Initiation of the inflammatory response
- Overproduction of sebum
- Hyperkeratinisation of cells
- Colonisation of p.acnes bacteria.

Initiation of the inflammatory response: New research shows that acne is caused by more than just blocked pores and bacteria—it's also about how the body's immune system reacts. A common skin bacterium called *Cutibacterium acnes* (or *P. acnes*) can trigger an immune reaction by waking up something called the inflammasome, which leads to the release of IL-1β. This potent chemical causes redness and swelling. This happens near the oil glands and hair follicles—where acne starts. The body also uses Toll-like receptors (TLRs) to sense bacteria. In acne, a specific TLR called TLR2 becomes more active and causes more inflammation. Some strains of *P. acnes* are worse than others at triggering this.

Besides this first-line defence, another part of the immune system called Th17 cells gets involved. These cells release IL-17, another chemical that makes inflammation worse. Researchers have found IL-17 in early acne spots, showing it plays a role right from the start. Interestingly, vitamin A and vitamin D can help reduce this response, which may explain why they work in acne treatments.

In summary, acne inflammation involves several parts of the immune system—not just bacteria and oil. Essential players include IL-1β, IL-17, TLR2, and the inflammasome. Understanding this could lead to better treatments that calm the immune system, rather than just treating the surface. More studies are still needed, but these findings give hope for new ways to treat acne more effectively.

Overproduction of sebum: Sebum is an oil produced by the sebaceous glands in the skin, which are prevalent all over the face. Acne is characterised by an overproduction of this oil, which is made up of lipids such as triglycerides, cholesterol, squalene and wax esters. Sebum has a natural benefit to hydrate and create a protective barrier on the skin's surface, but in excess, it can lead to issues such as breakouts. This increased oil can be visible on the face (especially the T-zone), becoming increasingly shiny throughout the day, makeup not staying in place and an increase in raised red pustules.

Hyperkeratinisation of cells: One of the earliest steps in acne development is hyperkeratinisation, which means too many skin cells build up inside hair follicles. Micromedones develop, which are clogged pores full of sebum and dead skin cells. Over time, these progress into open comedones (blackheads) and closed comedones (whiteheads).

Thickening of the keratin lining and subsequent obstruction of the sebaceous duct result in closed comedones (whiteheads) or open comedones (blackheads). The exact cause of this cell buildup is still being studied, but several factors are known to play a role. A chemical messenger in the skin, IL-1α, can cause skin cells to stick together and multiply, leading to clogged follicles. Changes in proteins like filaggrin and keratins K6 and K16 also suggest that skin cells are growing and maturing abnormally. Hormones, especially DHT, can worsen this problem by making skin cells in the follicles grow too fast. Low levels of linoleic acid (an essential fatty acid) and inevitable by-products in sebum (skin oil) may also trigger this process.

The bacteria P. acnes may contribute to forming micro-comedones, too. In some rare conditions like nevus comedonicus or Apert syndrome, mutations in the FGFR2 gene (especially Ser252Trp) cause overactive signals in the skin, leading to abnormal follicle development and acne. This mutation also increases IL-1α levels. Finally, some researchers think that inflammation may even start before the clogging begins.

Altogether, acne begins with clogged follicles caused by a mix of abnormal cell growth, hormones, and inflammation (Kurokawa et al., 2009).

Colonisation of p.acnes bacteria: The role of *P. acnes* (now called *Cutibacterium acnes*) in causing acne is still debated because it's a regular part of the skin's natural bacteria. However, new research into its genetic makeup has raised more questions about whether certain types of *P. acnes* might contribute to acne. Some studies show that P. acnes can trigger skin cells to release inflammatory signals and antimicrobial peptides, which are part of the body's natural defence system.

Interestingly, there are different types (or strains) of *P. acnes*, which don't all act the same way. Some strains seem to trigger stronger immune reactions than others, especially by increasing a molecule called hBD-2 in skin cells. While hBD-2 doesn't directly kill *P. acnes*, it works together with other natural antimicrobial substances, like cathelicidin and specific skin lipids, to help protect the skin.

Even in healthy skin, these antimicrobial peptides are present without any signs of redness or swelling. This suggests that they can be produced without causing inflammation, and that our normal skin bacteria might help keep this defence system active in a healthy way. In fact, some *P. acnes* strains might be helpful by boosting the skin's defences rather than causing harm.

Suppose scientists can identify P. acnes proteins that increase the skin's protective responses without triggering inflammation. In that case, we may be able to use that knowledge to prevent acne by strengthening the skin's natural barrier – stopping the harmful strains before they cause breakouts (Suh and Kwon, 2015).

Dysbiosis, the process leading to a disturbed skin barrier and disequilibrium of the cutaneous microbiome, resulting in the proliferation of P. acnes strains, is another crucial process that triggers acne. P. acnes activates the innate immunity via the expression of protease activated receptors (PARs), tumour necrosis factor (TNF) α and toll-like receptors (TLRs), and the production of interferon (INF) γ, interleukins (IL-8, IL12, IL-1), TNF, and matrix metalloproteinases (MMPs) by keratinocytes, resulting in the hyperkeratinisation of the pilosebaceous unit. Rebalancing the natural microbiome of the skin by restoring the natural skin barrier, limiting the proliferation of P. acnes on the skin by using topical antibacterials that do not cause resistance and regulating the quantity and quality of sebum will be the main acne treatment challenges in the future. The aim is to provide an update on the involvement of the sebaceous gland, the innate immunity and the cutaneous microbiome, how all of these factors promote acne, and to illustrate their links with current and future treatments.

TYPES OF ACNE

- Comedonal acne
- Inflammatory acne
- Nodulocystic acne
- Hormonal acne
- Fungal acne

Comedonal acne is often known as blackheads and white-heads.

Blackhead: Is characterised by a black bulge in the skin containing dead skin cells and sebum. The black colour is due to the oxidation of lipids. This is a non-inflamed blocked pore.

Whiteheads, also known as pimples, are inflammatory pustules with a white or yellow liquid enclosed in the pore.

Inflammatory acne: Papules and pustules.

Papules/papules: When inflammation is deep, this can cause pustules, which are an accumulation of pus in the pore alongside erythema and oedema (swelling).

Nodulystic acne: AKA nodules.

Nodules: Characterised by a papule with extensive inflammation deep within the skin that can be painful. This type of acne causes significant damage and inflammation, often resulting in scarring. It is essential not to try to pick any acne, but especially this type, as it's not possible to remove all of the buildup of pus and will only lead to further infection, inflammation and scarring.

<u>Hormonal acne</u>: An increase in androgens such as testosterone and a surge in the production of sebum often cause acne flare-ups in teenage years. Oestrogen (female sex hormone) affects oil glands by reducing the production of sebum. This is usually why men experience more acne than women. That's why, after menopause, when women's oestrogen levels begin to drop, sebum production may increase in some women, leading to breakouts.

Women's hormone levels fluctuate significantly throughout the monthly menstrual cycle, contributing to the highs and lows of different hormones. The increase in progesterone pre-period is a large contributor to breakouts along the chin and jawline during this time.

<u>Fungal acne</u>: Fungal acne is an infection present within the hair follicles, creating small clusters of itchy red bumps filled with pus. This is caused by a fungus called Malassezia yeast. Although acne vulgaris (regular acne) and fungal acne can look similar, a distant difference between the two is that fungal acne is itchy. Both types of acne can be present on someone's face in different areas at the same time. This is most likely to occur in humid climates, among clients who sweat excessively (hyperhidrosis), those with a weakened

immune system, and individuals who use oil-based moisturisers and sunscreens.

COMMON ACNE TRIGGERS

Hormones: Androgenic hormones increase the size of the
sebaceous glands and the amount of sebum in both female
and male adolescents. Androgen levels may be normal,
but a correlation of increased sensitivity to the androgen
hormones is common.

Polycystic ovarian syndrome: PCOS is a condition characterised by an overproduction of androgens (male sex
hormones), resulting in multiple cysts developing in the
ovaries. Insulin resistance is common in people with PCOS,
and this can manifest as acne on the skin.

Occlusion: There are many ways that occlusive breakouts
occur. This could be due to wearing a tight hat or helmet in
a warm climate where you get sweaty. And this pressure and
sebum can result in a pustule.

Stress and cortisol: When we are stressed, our autonomic
nervous system increases the amount of cortisol within our
body. Hormones involved with the body's stress response
can also stimulate sebaceous glands to produce more oil.
Stress increases the level of inflammation in the body
and can impair the body's natural antimicrobial defences,

throwing the microbiome off.

Medications: Contraceptives are artificial hormones used to alter our cycle to prevent pregnancy. However, depending on our baseline hormone levels, this can either disrupt the balance of various hormones, leading to more breakouts, or balance our hormones and improve our skin. This depends on the type of contraceptive and your individual levels, so you may need to try a few different kinds before finding the one that works best for you and your skin.

Skincare products: Some skincare products can throw out the skin's pH balance or disrupt the barrier, resulting in breakouts. Ingredients such as vitamin A (retinol), AHAs, or BHA's (Glycolic acid) are effective in balancing oil production in the skin and promoting cell turnover. However, when used in excess (in frequency or strength %), they can lead to over-exfoliation of the skin.

Some ultra-hydrating skincare products, which use oils and occlusives, can suffocate pores and add extra oil, potentially worsening acne.

Diet: Multiple studies have demonstrated the connection between high GI (glycaemic index), sugar and dairy diets and how they result in the production and aggravation of acne. Diets high in these types of foods produce a higher level of insulin and inflammation in the skin, which is a contributor to acne.

Other studies have also shown the benefits of consuming omega-3 fatty acids from healthy fish and oils, leading to a better balance of oils and fewer, less aggravated breakouts.

Recent research on the effects of probiotics on the skin's microbiome has shown positive effects (Baldwin and Tan, 2020).

ACNE MYTHS & MISINFORMATION

"Acne is caused by dirty skin"

Although dirt can be a contributor to breakouts, having acne does not mean that someone is dirty. As we know, it is a combination of excess oil production, over keratinization of cells, hormones and inflammation in the skin. Simply cleaning the skin is not enough to resolve acne.

"You should dry acne out"

It used to be common for people to try to dry out acne with ingredients like alcohol and benzyl peroxide. Although it may give temporary improvement, doing so can dehydrate the skin and throw off the skin microbiome, resulting in further breakouts.

"Scrubbing gets rid of pimples"

Excessive scrubbing or the use of physical exfoliants on breakouts can cause multiple issues. The rough surface can cause microtears in the skin, which may result in the spread of further breakouts. Excessive scrubbing can also unbalance the skin microbiome.

"Sunscreen causes breakouts"

Sunscreen is an essential and non-negotiable step of the skin care routine for all. If someone is breaking out from their sunscreen, it's likely due to how the brand or product interacts with their skin, so they should try an alternate brand.

PROFESSIONAL ACNE TREATMENTS

Initial consultation: This first appointment starts with a skin analysis. We ask a lot of questions about your usual routine and habits, as well as how your skin reacts and responds in different situations. We conduct an in-depth health assessment, which includes inquiring about your previous medical history, any medications you are currently taking, past allergies or reactions, and any factors that may contraindicate treatment.

In-clinic options:

Chemical peels: This treatment involves cleansing and preparing your skin before applying an acid to exfoliate, encouraging cell turnover. There are various acids we can use that will affect the skin in different ways.

Salicylic acid is best suited for acne-prone skin. Reduces oil production while encouraging cell turnover to unblock pores and reduce oil secretion.

Glycolic acid is best suited for aging skin. This is going to decrease the appearance of fine lines, even skin tone (pigmentation) and encourage cell turnover to leave us with a brighter, tighter complexion.

Lactic acid is best suited for aged skin. This peel encourages cell turnover, leaving skin smoother and more refined.

Mandelic acid: Best for acne-prone skin. This acid reduces sebum production, encourages cell turnover, and dissolves sebum in the pores.

Modified Jessner Peel: One of my all-time favourite peels, as it is a supercharged all-rounder that seems to be able to do everything. With the combination of salicylic acid, lactic acid and resorcinol or citric acid, it can tackle all concerns such as signs of ageing, pigmentation and acne.

LED LIGHT THERAPY (BLUE/RED LIGHT):

A light-emitting device that focuses on encouraging wound healing, stimulating collagen and elastin production and, in the case of a blue light, killing bacteria on the skin. There are varying lights that can be chosen on the LED for different benefits:

- **Red:** Stimulated collagen and elastin
- **Yellow:** Promotes wound healing and decreases bruising.
- **Blue:** Kills bacteria on the skin that contribute to acne.
- **Green:** Assists with decreasing pigmentation

Micro needling: Once the breakouts are well under control, the implementation of Fractional RF is encouraged to smooth skin texture, reduce scarring and reduce pigmentation. This treatment combines tiny needles with heat to stimulate tissue regeneration and promote the production of collagen and elastin in the skin.

Prescriptions: If in-clinic treatments have been given a good go and are not proving to be effective for the client, then they may seek further assistance from their GP or dermatologist, who may choose to prescribe antibiotics, topical tretinoin cream, or acne medication to decrease the severity and frequency of lesions. These treatments can be effective but come with risks, so it is essential to discuss them thoroughly with your doctor before commencing to decide what is right for you.

Laser/IPL for post-acne pigmentation: these treatments are effective in resurfacing the skin post-acne. They directly benefit post-inflammatory hyperpigmentation and scarring by resurfacing the skin and encouraging the growth of healthy new tissue.

It is essential for the treating practitioner to thoroughly assess the client's barrier before any in-clinic treatments or skincare prescription. This is because if the barrier is not functioning correctly, it will not respond appropriately to treatments, and can result in worsening of the condition. If the barrier appears impaired, it is essential to nourish the skin with probiotics for the microbiome and simple, non-irritating skincare to balance the skin, before trying to resurface.

AT-HOME SKINCARE FOR ACNE-PRONE SKIN

Professional treatments are complemented by high-performance skincare. Here's what I recommend for my acne-prone clients:

Cleanser:

Medik8 gentle foaming cleanser

A mild foaming wash infused with rosemary, designed to remove dirt, makeup, and impurities without disrupting the skin's balance. Removes oil without leaving the skin feeling tight.

Probiotics:

Dermiotic

A daily elixir fortified with pre- and postbiotics to balance the skin's microbiome, which assists in calming the skin and improving barrier function.

Hydration:

Niacinamide (vitamin B):

A hydration serum designed to improve skin barrier function, reduce breakouts, and alleviate congestion by regulating oil flow.

Resurfacers:

Medik8 Crystal Retinal

Vitamin A is critical for cell turnover, fine line reduction, and reducing oil production and clarity. Retinaldehyde is a potent, but gentler, alternative to prescription retinoids.

OR

Exfol-X

An AHA and BHA serum that brightens and exfoliates your skin to reduce the appearance of hyperpigmentation, decongest pores and improve skin texture.

Hydrating SPF: Uberzinc

A lightweight physical sunscreen with the benefits of zinc to lightly hydrate your skin and provide sun protection.

*It is imperative to use sunscreen while using active

ingredients; if you don't, it might even make your skin look worse! As active ingredients work tirelessly to resurface your skin, they bring you a brighter, clearer complexion. "They remove the dead skin on the surface to reveal newer skin underneath. However, this newer skin is more susceptible to burning and accelerated aging. So very important to keep it protected, otherwise you could end up looking older.

Special Treatments:

- **Clay mask:** A weekly treatment that is beneficial to absorb excess oil from your skin, leaving you feeling clean and fresh. Ensure to hydrate after this treatment so it doesn't over-dry your skin and only use as directed.

It is essential to start with a simple routine of cleanser, moisturiser and sunscreen, then slowly add in extra steps to reduce the amount of stress on your skin. It takes time to see the results, so don't rush it. It may take at least 3 months for you to start really seeing the results, so this is not a time to be impatient. It's essential to give products a fair trial over several months, rather than changing them after a week of no results, as they take time. This constant change may further disrupt the skin's barrier.

ACNE SCARRING & PIGMENTATION

Once acne has cleared, unfortunately, we are left with the evidence of what once was, including pigmentation and acne scarring. Post-inflammatory hyperpigmentation (PIHP) can be visible as dark spots on the skin that are leftover once a pustule has healed. Similarly occurring, post-inflammatory erythema is a red spot that is left over afterwards. The more inflammatory a breakout is and whether it is picked, plays a large part in whether a scar is left in the skin. Formation of scar tissue can occur when a breakout that has been inflamed for a long time or has been picked at or squeezed results in a wound that turns into a scar. Scarring should only be treated once all acne lesions are controlled and the inflammation in the skin has decreased.

Effective treatments for scarring include micro-needling, lasers, Peels, and PRP. These treatments work to encourage cell turnover, promoting the growth of healthy new cells. This results in a brighter and clearer complexion.

4

Embracing the Change – Menopause

Menopause is often discussed in hushed tones, as if it marks the end of something: youth, vibrancy, or beauty. But for many women I see in clinic, it's not about age, but about control. Control over how they feel in their skin, how they show up in the world, and how they recognise themselves in the mirror. And when that sense of control starts to slip, whether due to skin changes, mood fluctuations, or a loss of confidence, it can feel deeply personal.

This chapter isn't here to promise a fountain of youth or offer miracle cures. Instead, it's about understanding what's happening—hormonally, structurally, and emotionally— and offering tools to support your skin and self through this significant life shift. Whether you're perimenopausal, postmenopausal, or somewhere in between, this chapter is a roadmap to feeling informed and empowered.

HORMONES & SKIN: THE CONNECTION YOU CAN'T IGNORE

The skin is our body's largest organ, and it responds promptly to hormonal changes. Think back to puberty—the first time most of us noticed the relationship between hormones and our complexion. Menopause is another critical milestone, often with just as many visible changes.

The transition typically occurs across four overlapping stages:

1. Premenopause
This is the baseline phase before symptoms begin. Hormone levels are considered "normal," though subtle shifts in estrogen and progesterone may start in the mid-to-late 30s. Some women notice a gradual increase in skin dryness or irregular breakouts at this time, even before periods become irregular.

2. Perimenopause
It usually begins in the early 40s, but it can start earlier. It's a turbulent period marked by fluctuating estrogen and progesterone levels. These shifts cause hot flashes, mood swings, night sweats, and yes—dramatic changes in the skin. You may notice dry patches one week, oiliness the next. Skin may become reactive, sensitive, or unpredictable.

3. Menopause

Officially diagnosed when you haven't had a period for 12 months. Estrogen production drops significantly, and many symptoms intensify. The loss of estrogen impacts collagen production, skin hydration, wound healing, and elasticity. It's the most common time for women to notice wrinkles becoming more prominent, cheeks losing volume, and pigmentation worsening.

4. Postmenopause

This is the new normal. Hormone levels remain low and steady. While some symptoms subside, skin may continue to thin, sag, or dull if not actively supported.

WHY ESTROGEN MATTERS

Estrogen plays a critical role in maintaining the youthful qualities of skin. It promotes collagen and elastin synthesis, supports barrier function, regulates melanin production, and improves hydration by increasing hyaluronic acid levels. As estrogen declines, we begin to see:

- **Reduced collagen:** Up to 30% loss in the first five years post-menopause
- **Thinner epidermis:** Skin becomes fragile and slow to repair
- **Dehydration:** Less hyaluronic acid leads to dullness, dryness, and increased fine lines

- **Hyperpigmentation:** Fluctuations in melanin-stimulating hormones can trigger melasma or sunspots
- **Increased sensitivity:** A compromised barrier leads to redness, irritation, and rosacea-like symptoms

And that's just from estrogen. A drop in progesterone can throw off the oil balance of the skin—causing either flakiness or unexpected breakouts. Meanwhile, testosterone and other androgens may become relatively more dominant, causing issues like jawline acne or facial hair growth (hello unexpected chin hair?!).

SKIN CHANGES YOU MIGHT NOTICE

No two women experience menopause the same way, but the patterns are common. You might recognise some of these signs:

- Wrinkles deepen due to collagen loss
- Skin becomes thinner and more fragile
- Jawline begins to soften or sag
- Dry patches or dullness take longer to recover
- Pigmentation darkens and becomes stubborn
- Skin feels itchy, tight, or sensitive
- Breakouts or oiliness despite previous dryness
- Redness and broken capillaries appear more frequently
- Neck and décolletage may show signs of aging faster than the face

These changes are not simply cosmetic; they can impact your confidence, your sense of self, and how comfortable you feel in your skin.

STRESS, SLEEP & SKIN RESILIENCE

One of the lesser-discussed elements of menopause is the increase in cortisol, the body's primary stress hormone. Hormonal shifts during this time can increase cortisol production, especially if sleep becomes disrupted or anxiety heightens. Elevated cortisol depletes skin barrier lipids, weakens immune function, and contributes to inflammatory skin conditions like rosacea, eczema, and adult acne.

Sleep disturbances are also common due to night sweats, hot flashes, or mood changes. But sleep is when your body repairs itself, including your skin. Poor quality sleep directly affects skin hydration, cell turnover, and the skin's ability to recover from environmental stressors.

A regular wind-down routine, reduced screen time, cool bedroom temperatures, and natural supplements like magnesium or glycine may support more restful sleep. And this, in turn, helps the skin remain resilient.

THE ROLE OF OXIDATIVE STRESS IN MENOPAUSAL SKIN

Oxidative stress is one of the most critical internal contributors to aging, and it becomes increasingly relevant in menopause. It refers to the imbalance between free radicals (unstable molecules produced by pollution, UV rays, stress, alcohol, and even digestion) and your body's ability to neutralise them with antioxidants.

With declining estrogen, your skin's natural antioxidant defences drop too. This means:
- Collagen is broken down faster
- Pigmentation worsens due to melanocyte damage
- Skin tone becomes uneven
- Wrinkles form more easily
- Skin may feel rough or look sallow

Combatting oxidative stress involves both topical antioxidants and dietary support. Think vitamin C serums, niacinamide, green tea extract—and internally, foods rich in colour (berries, spinach, turmeric, matcha, nuts, seeds).

PROFESSIONAL TREATMENTS TO SUPPORT MIDLIFE SKIN

While we can't stop time, we *can* support the skin's natural processes with treatments designed to strengthen, hydrate, and rebuild.

At Skin Societé, we offer a range of dermal therapies suited to menopausal and postmenopausal skin. Here's how they help:

SKIN NEEDLING (COLLAGEN INDUCTION THERAPY)

Microneedling uses controlled micro-injuries to stimulate the production of collagen and elastin. It's ideal for fine lines, texture, pigmentation, and overall rejuvenation.

RADIOFREQUENCY SKIN TIGHTENING

A gentle yet effective treatment that utilises heat energy to stimulate the dermal layers, thereby enhancing firmness, elasticity, and jawline definition. Great for those seeing early signs of sagging.

FRACTIONAL RF

Combines microneedling and radiofrequency to address skin laxity, enlarged pores, and fine lines. It's especially effective on the neck, cheeks, and around the mouth—areas often impacted by estrogen loss.

LASER TREATMENTS

We offer medical-grade lasers that target pigmentation, redness, and vascular lesions without harming surrounding tissue. Our approach is tailored and gentle, especially for sensitive, mature skin.

- **Laser facials:** For overall tone and redness
- **Vascular laser:** To reduce visible capillaries and facial flushing
- **Pigment laser:** To fade melasma, sunspots, and uneven tone

ENZYME AND CHEMICAL PEELS

We use medical-grade, evidence-based peels that gently exfoliate and brighten the skin. Regular peels promote cellular turnover, lighten pigmentation, and reduce pore size. This is especially helpful when hormones slow skin renewal.

At Skin Societé, these are often integrated into our monthly membership plans, so clients stay consistent and achieve long-term skin goals.

AT-HOME SKINCARE: THE DAILY RITUALS THAT MATTER

Supporting menopausal skin from home is essential. With the proper skincare, you can significantly reduce the impact of hormonal decline. Here's what I personally recommend to my clients:

CLEANSER: MEDIK8 LIPID-BALANCE CLEANSING OIL

A nourishing cleanser that gently removes makeup, sunscreen, and impurities without stripping the skin. It supports your lipid barrier, leaving the skin soft and supple, not tight.

HYDRATION SERUM: HYALAVIVE

A deeply hydrating serum with multiple molecular weights of hyaluronic acid. Formulated with ceramides and B12, it targets inflammation and dryness, two hallmarks of menopausal skin.

ANTIOXIDANTS: EFFICA C OR SYNERGIE SUPER SERUM

These potent serums protect against environmental damage, support collagen production, and improve tone. Vitamin C is particularly effective at fading pigmentation and boosting radiance.

VITAMIN A: MEDIK8 CRYSTAL RETINAL

A game changer for menopausal skin. Retinaldehyde is gentler than prescription retinoids but still highly effective at boosting cell turnover, reducing fine lines, and clearing congestion.

MOISTURISER: RECLAIM ANTI-AGEING MOIS-TURISER

Formulated with peptides, antioxidants, and marine actives. It firms, calms, and restores skin overnight while helping to rebuild collagen.

SPF: MEDIK8 ADVANCED DAY TOTAL PROTECT SPF 30

Daily sun protection is non-negotiable. This SPF shields against UV, infrared, and environmental aggressors, while maintaining hydration and preventing further pigmentation.

SPECIAL TREATMENTS:

- **Night Eye Cream:** Targets puffiness, darkness, and crow's feet.

- **Mask Erase:** An overnight, collagen-boosting mask to plump and brighten dull skin.

INTERNAL WELLNESS = EXTERNAL RADIANCE

Menopause is a full-body experience, and supporting skin health means taking care of everything below the surface, too.

- Stay hydrated - Aim for 2–3 litres of water per day.
- Prioritise protein - Collagen is a protein, and your body needs adequate intake to rebuild tissue.
- Balance your gut - Probiotics and prebiotic foods (like yoghurt, kimchi, oats, garlic) support digestion, hormone metabolism, and skin clarity.
- Supplement wisely - Speak to your GP or naturopath about omega-3s, magnesium, collagen peptides, or adaptogens if you're feeling run down.
- Move your body - Exercise supports lymphatic flow, circulation, hormone balance, and sleep quality.

FINAL THOUGHTS: THIS IS A BEGINNING, NOT AN END

Menopause is not a loss. It's a transition—a time to pause, reflect, and reorient toward your own care. Yes, your skin may feel different. But with the proper knowledge, treatments, and support, it can feel stronger, calmer, and more radiant than ever.

At Skin Societé, we understand this journey intimately. We don't chase trends or offer band-aid fixes. We partner with you through the changes, offering education, high-performance skincare, and safe, effective treatments tailored to your evolving needs.

Because you deserve to feel good in your skin. At every age. Through every season. And especially now.

5

Pigmentation

WHAT IS PIGMENTATION?

The number of melanocytes and melanin present in the skin determines the colour and clarity of our skin. Increased pigmentation, also known as hyperpigmentation, develops when there is a higher concentration of melanin and/or melanocytes in the skin, resulting in a patch of darker skin. This can result in skin appearing to have uneven skin colouring as some areas are darker or lighter than others. In some cases, pigment can be lost from the skin, resulting in hypopigmentation (white patches). A decrease in melanin synthesis or a reduction in melanocytes causes this. Melanin is a natural pigment produced by melanocyte cells, which colours our hair, skin, and eyes. The main factor that contributes to our colouring is the quantity of melanin. Other factors include carotenoids and haemoglobin. Melanin plays a vital role in protecting us from ultraviolet light (UV). Our skin is repeatedly exposed to UV radiation, which is a significant stressor to our skin and can lead to skin cancer from excessive exposure. The melanin within our skin does a great job at absorbing UV light to reduce the impact on our surrounding cells, but melanin also has antioxidant and radical scavenging properties.

Pigmentation is one of the most common concerns that our clients come to us with. They are concerned about freckles, sunspots and melasma, all of which create a variation in the colour of their skin. This is something we can aim to improve with the use of at-home skincare and in-clinic treatments. Although pigmentation is often known to be a recurring issue if the melanocyte is retriggered, it is usually a lifelong journey to keep it at bay.

HOW PIGMENT IS PRODUCED

Melanogenesis is the biological process through which melanin, the pigment responsible for skin, hair, and eye colour, is produced. This process takes place in specialised cells called melanocytes, which are in the basal layer of the epidermis, the bottom layer of the skin. Melanogenesis plays a critical role not only in determining skin tone but also in protecting the skin from damage caused by ultraviolet (UV) radiation.

Melanocytes in the Basal Layer

Melanocytes are dendritic (branch-like) cells positioned

between the basal keratinocytes in the epidermis. They originate from neural crest cells during embryonic development. Although melanocytes only make up about 1 in every 10 basal cells, they play an essential role in pigmentation. Each melanocyte is associated with approximately 30 to 40 neighbouring keratinocytes, forming what is called the epidermal-melanin unit.

These melanocytes produce melanin within specialised intracellular organelles called melanosomes. The primary function of melanocytes is to synthesise melanin and distribute it to keratinocytes, where it provides pigmentation and acts as a natural sunscreen by absorbing and scattering harmful UV rays.

Tyrosinase Enzyme Activity

The production of melanin begins inside the melanocytes with the activation of the enzyme tyrosinase, which is the key regulatory enzyme in melanogenesis. Tyrosinase is a copper-dependent enzyme that catalyses the initial steps of melanin synthesis. Its activity is the rate-limiting step of melanogenesis, meaning that if tyrosinase is inhibited, melanin production decreases significantly.

The melanogenesis pathway starts when the amino acid tyrosine is converted by tyrosinase into dopaquinone. From this point, the process can follow two primary pathways depending on the type of melanin being produced:

- **Eumelanin**, the brown-black pigment, provides strong UV protection.
- **Pheomelanin**, the red-yellow pigment, offers less UV protection and is more common in lighter skin tones and red hair.

Eumelanin production continues through several enzymatic reactions that polymerize dopaquinone into dense, dark pigment granules. Tyrosinase and related enzymes such as TRP-1 and TRP-2 (tyrosinase-related proteins) are involved in this complex synthesis process.

Transfer of Melanin to Keratinocytes

Once melanin is produced and packaged into melanosomes, the next critical step is the transfer of these pigment-containing melanosomes from the melanocytes to the surrounding keratinocytes. This transfer occurs through the dendritic extensions of the melanocytes, which reach up between multiple keratinocytes in the basal and suprabasal layers.

The keratinocytes engulf the melanosomes through a process called phagocytosis, where the dendritic tips deliver melanosomes into the keratinocytes. Once inside, the melanosomes migrate to position themselves above the keratinocyte nucleus, forming a protective cap. This cap shields the DNA from UV-induced damage by absorbing and scattering UV radiation.

The efficiency and quantity of melanosome transfer play a significant role in visible skin colour. Darker skin tones are not due to more melanocytes but rather to larger, more densely pigmented melanosomes that are distributed individually within keratinocytes. In contrast, lighter skin tones have smaller, less pigmented melanosomes that tend to cluster and degrade more quickly.

How Pigment Appears at the Surface

As keratinocytes gradually move upward from the basal layer toward the skin surface (a process known as keratinocyte differentiation and turnover), they carry the melanin-containing melanosomes with them. Over about 28 days, keratinocytes migrate through the different layers of the epidermis, from the basal layer to the stratum corneum.

When the keratinocytes reach the outermost layer of the skin, the stratum corneum, they become flattened, dead skin cells (corneocytes) but still retain the melanin within them. This deposited melanin gives the skin its surface colour. The final appearance of pigment on the skin depends on several factors, including the amount of melanin produced, the size and distribution of melanosomes, and the rate of skin turnover.

Sun exposure increases melanogenesis by stimulating melanocytes through UV radiation, particularly UVB, which activates tyrosinase and other signalling pathways, leading to tanning. Conversely, as keratinocytes shed naturally through exfoliation, pigment gradually fades unless continually stimulated.

In summary, melanogenesis begins with melanocytes in the basal layer producing melanin through tyrosinase-driven pathways. Melanin is packaged into melanosomes, transferred to keratinocytes, and eventually appears at the skin surface as keratinocytes migrate upwards. This process is vital for pigmentation and essential for protecting the skin from UV-induced damage.

TYPES OF PIGMENTATION

Post-Inflammatory Hyperpigmentation (PIH)

This is pigmentation that develops in an area of skin following inflammation or injury. This may include chemical exposure, burns, wounds, psoriasis, atopic dermatitis or acne. The delayed inflammation results in discolouration of the skin, making it look darker after it has healed. During its formation, the skin synthesises a higher rate of melanin. PIHP is more common in darker skin tones (or also known as a darker Fitzpatrick score) due to the larger saturation of free melanin present in the skin. PIHP is an adverse reaction to a treatment and is not considered a normal response. This is more likely to occur if the wrong treatment, of too high a strength, is given to a patient who hasn't had the appropriate prep and/or aftercare. This is why it is essential to have a thorough skin analysis completed with a professional who is educated in skin care and dermal therapies.

Melasma

Melasma is recognised as one of the most challenging types of pigmentation to treat, primarily because of the multiple factors contributing to its formation and its deep-seated location in the skin layers. Melasma is brown, grey-toned pigmentation that develops on a person's face or arms. It may be genetic, but sun exposure, prolonged heat, pregnancy, hormones, and contraception can all be factors to bring it on. Its slang term is "pregnancy mask" due to the frequency of this occurring during pregnancy in a butterfly mask shape along the forehead, cheeks and upper lip.

Sun Damage

Sun damage, also known as solar lentigines, are age spots or liver spots that appear on the face after many years of sun exposure and, in most cases, inadequate sun protection. They are a result of the accumulation of UV exposure, resulting in a brown mark on the skin. They are often present on the sides of the face, neck and decolletage.

Freckles

Freckles, also known as ephelides, are small brown and/or

orange dots of pigment across a person's skin. They can be present all over the body, and the depth in colour, number, and placement can be dependent on genetic factors, sun exposure, and sun protection. People who are predisposed to having freckles may notice an increase in the number and depth of colour after periods of long-term sun exposure. They are often most prominent on the face, decolletage and arms. This is more common in people with fair skin or a light Fitzpatrick skin type.

Hypopigmentation

Hypopigmentation is the absence of pigment in the skin. This is the opposite result of hyperpigmentation but can often be caused by a lot of the same factors, such as trauma and inflammation. But it can also be caused by the medical condition vitiligo. This condition is characterised by macules of a white chalky substance on the skin and melanin loss, causing white patches on the skin.

PIGMENTATION TRIGGERS

- UV exposure: This is the most common cause. UVA and UVB promote the production of pigmentation in the skin.
- Heat: Pigmentation can be triggered by prolonged exposure to heat, so the risk is increased in people who live in hot climates, work in heat-related

occupations, use saunas and heat therapy and work out a lot.

- <u>Hormonal fluctuations</u>: Hormonal changes during pregnancy, from contraception or during menopause can all contribute to pigmentation.
- <u>Inflammation</u>: delayed wound healing or picking of acne can result in prolonged inflammation, Pigment from PIHP, infection and possibly scarring.
- Certain medications or cosmetics:

THE FITZPATRICK SKIN TYPE SCALE

The Fitzpatrick score is a scale used during skin assessments to determine the colour of a person's skin. It is a score from 1 to 6 that assesses how much melanin pigment is present in the skin and the effect of exposure to ultraviolet light and radiation (tanning). Pale skin is more prone to burning, whereas darker skin has more melanin to absorb the UV rays, making it less likely to burn and less severely.

Fitzpatrick scale:

		1	2	3	4	5	6
Skin Type		Skin Type I	Skin Type II	Skin Type III	Skin Type IV	Skin Type V	Skin Type VI
Skin Color		Light, pale white	White, fair	Medium, white to olive	Beige-olive, moderate brown	Brown, dark brown	Very dark brown to black
Reaction to Sunburn		Always burns	Usually burns	Sometimes mild burns	Rarely burns	Very rarely burns	Never burns
Reaction to Sun Tanning		Never tans	Tans with difficulty	Gradually tans to olive	Easy tans to moderate brown	Tans very easily	Always tans
Skin Cancer Risk		Greatest risk	High risk	High risk	At risk	Relatively rare	Relatively rare

Falinski, J. (2024). *Fitzpatrick Scale and Skin Types.* [online] Clinilabs | The CRO for CNS. Available at: https://clinilabs. com/volunteers/fp/.

Darker Fitzpatrick scores are at higher risk of developing PIHP, so it is essential to consider this when treatment planning. Always start with the lowest strength of resurfacing treatments before gradually building up. Be cautious with lasers, and it is essential to make sure a test patch is completed in the area before any treatments.

PROFESSIONAL TREATMENT OPTIONS

Chemical peels: These are a great way to remove pigmentation gently. Lighter Fitzpatrick types can progress more quickly through the strengths of peels to achieve a result more quickly, while darker skin tones require more caution. Chemical peels work by inhibiting the tyrosinase in the skin to reduce pigmentation. They also work by resurfacing the skin to remove pigmented cells from the surface, to reveal brighter skin underneath. It is crucial to avoid picking at or pulling the skin after a peel, as this can lead to PIHP and scarring.

Peels that benefit clients with pigmentation concerns include:

Lactic acid: a large molecule, a slow-penetrating BHA peel that often has minimal downtime. It is excellent to brighten and lighten the skin, improving the appearance of fine lines and wrinkles.

Mandelic acid: Promoted cell turnover to help fade dark patches, resulting in a more uniform complexion over time.

Azelaic acid: A tyrosinase inhibitor that helps to reduce pigmentation. This is particularly beneficial for individuals with darker Fitzpatrick skin types and those experiencing persistent spots from PIHP and melasma.

TCA: A very strong and powerful peel that has the power to lift deep pigmentation. However, the skin must be adequately prepped to prevent further damage. In some cases, this peel can lift to 90% of pigment in one session, although with serious results comes serious downtime. The strict aftercare regime must be adhered to prevent reappearance or worsening of pigment. This is not suitable for darker Fitzpatrick scores.

Laser treatments: A laser can be used to specifically target the pigmentation in the skin, which absorbs the light, so the surrounding skin remains unaffected. The laser heats the pigment immediately, causing it to shatter and become less dense. As macrophages in the skin clean up this debris, the skin becomes clearer and brighter.

Laser toning is a standard method used to treat melasma by effectively reducing the size and pigment in coloured lesions. It is recommended to have 3-4 sessions around 1 month apart to allow the skin to heal in between. Results can take up to 3-6 months post-initiating treatment to show. However, follow-up sessions may be required, as it's common for the pigment to result post-laser.

IPL is a beneficial treatment for freckles because it uses broad light to cover a larger surface area, making it more effective.

Micro needling: Although laser and chemical peels will do the groundwork for most of the deeper pigment, once it reaches the surface, skin needling can be added to the mix. Skin needling uses multiple small needles in the skin to cause an inflammatory response that stimulates the production of collagen and elastin. It is beneficial for encouraging the growth of healthy new, resilient skin and is an excellent end-stage treatment for PIHP and superficial pigmentation. For clients with heat-induced pigmentation, I recommend caution and avoid RF, opting for standard skin needling instead, to prevent the device's heat from stimulating further pigmentation.

Pigmentation is very slow and difficult to treat, so it is essential to set realistic expectations of results and timelines with the client before starting treatment. As we know, pigmentation is caused by melanin, a naturally occurring protective mechanism that's present in our skin, so we can't get rid of it. Pigment is stored deep within your skin. Once transferred to keratinocytes, it takes approximately 28-40 days to turn over. Once melanocytes have been triggered, they can remain overactive for a long time, even after the initial trigger is gone. Over-aggressive treatments can worsen pigmentation by causing excessive inflammation in the skin, leading to poor wound healing and PIHP.

Sunscreen is a non-negotiable for all clients, but especially when trying to treat pigmentation. Why would you bother working so hard to remove pigmentation if you are not willing to prevent more from developing?

TOPICAL PIGMENT-FADING INGREDIENTS

Topical pigment-fading ingredients are essential for treating pigmentation by targeting multiple steps in the melanogenesis process. Tyrosinase inhibitors such as Vitamin C, Kojic acid, Azelaic acid, Niacinamide, Arbutin, and Licorice root work by blocking the enzyme tyrosinase, which is responsible for melanin production. This helps to prevent the formation of new pigment and gradually fades existing pigmentation.

Vitamin C is a powerful antioxidant that brightens skin and reduces oxidative stress by fighting free radicals.

Kojic acid not only inhibits tyrosinase but also has antibacterial properties.

Azelaic acid helps reduce inflammation and is particularly effective for post-inflammatory hyperpigmentation (PIHP).

Niacinamide strengthens the skin barrier and reduces pigment transfer from melanocytes to keratinocytes.

Arbutin is a natural derivative of hydroquinone that safely fades pigment.

Liquorice root contains liquiritin and glabridin, which soothe inflammation and lighten dark spots.

Retinoids speed up cell turnover, pushing pigmented cells to the surface faster and promoting the growth of fresh, evenly toned skin.

Tranexamic acid, both topical and oral, helps to reduce stubborn pigmentation like melasma by calming melanocyte overactivity and reducing vascular factors that trigger pigment. Together, these ingredients offer a robust, multi-pathway approach to achieving clearer, brighter skin.

THE ROLE OF SUNSCREEN

UV rays that can penetrate the ozone layer consist of long-wavelength radiation and are 320-400nm (nanometres). Only 5% of the radiation can pass through the ozone, which consists of UVB and UVC. There is increasing damage occurring to our ozone layer, which, over time, will affect the level of protection that we are receiving from the ozone layer. Scientists have determined that as small as a 1% reduction in the ozone layer can increase our skin cancer mortality rate by 1-2% (Brenner and Hearing, 2007). UVB is also more cytotoxic (cancer-causing) and mutagenic than UVA. Although UVB is unable to pass through glass, UVA can penetrate down to the dermal layer, where it has the most impact. It is found that up to 50% of UVA damage occurs while you are in the shade. UVB rays cause direct DNA damage, leading to mutations that can result in skin cancers like BCC and SCC. UVA causes indirect damage by creating harmful molecules called reactive oxygen species (ROS), which also harm DNA. Both UVA and UVB can create DNA lesions, but UVB is the leading cause. The body can repair some of the damage, but mutations in key genes like p53 can occur if repairs fail, increasing skin cancer risk.

This highlights the importance of protecting skin from both UVA and UVB.

The amount of damage that can occur because of UV damage is broad, so it is essential to wear a broad-spectrum sunscreen every day (yes, even when you are spending most of the day inside!). It is necessary to choose a sunscreen that is SPF 50+. It is beneficial to apply one teaspoon of your sunscreen first thing in the morning to minimise sun exposure before application and to reapply throughout the day. One teaspoon is regarded as the correct amount to ensure the best coverage. Keep in mind, this is only enough for your face. You also require one teaspoon per limb. To cover your whole body, you may need around seven teaspoons worth of sunscreen. It is recommended to reapply every 4 hours, unless you are engaging in physical exercise, sweating heavily, swimming, or any other activity that may dilute or wear away your sunscreen, reducing its ability to provide adequate coverage. When I first mention to my clients the importance of reapplication throughout the day, they tend to look at me like I'm crazy and say, "Jemma, I'm not going to apply sunscreen over my face of makeup", which I under-stand! But don't worry, other methods of application won't affect your makeup. Some brands offer mineral powder sunscreens that apply similarly to a setting powder, while others come in spritz versions that you can spray over your face to boost your sun protection.

There are various types of sunscreens available to us. So, it's essential to understand the different kinds to make an educated decision on the type you will use.

Chemical sunscreen

A chemical sunscreen works by absorbing the sun's rays, converting them to heat. ("Mineral Sunscreen Vs Chemical Sunscreen - La Roche-Posay") It has a lightweight texture and is easy to blend into the skin. A drawback of this is that it takes around 20 minutes post-application to provide full coverage to the skin.

Physical sunscreen

Physical, also known as mineral, sunscreens create a barrier or a "block" to reflect the sun's rays. It starts working immediately after being applied to the skin. However, it has a thicker texture and can leave a white cast on the skin.

Both chemical and physical sunscreens are effective in providing broad-spectrum sun protection. For clients concerned about pigmentation, I recommend a physical over a chemical sunscreen. This is due to the heat production from a chemical sunscreen, which can, in some cases, contribute to the worsening of pigment.

SPF ratings

I often hear a lot of debate around SPF ratings, and I am here to clear up the confusion surrounding these ratings and their expected levels of coverage. A sunscreen with an SPF rating of 30+ is estimated to filter 96.7% of UVB radiation. Whereas an SPF rating of 50 is estimated to filter 98% of UVB. So as long as at least one teaspoon of SPF is applied all over the area, both can provide adequate protection for your skin.

PIGMENTATION AND HORMONES

Hormones play a significant role in pigmentation, especially in hormonally driven conditions like melasma. Oestrogen and progesterone stimulate melanocyte activity, increasing melanin production. This is particularly evident during times of hormonal fluctuation, such as pregnancy, perimenopause, or with the use of oral contraceptives and hormone replacement therapy (HRT). Additionally, cortisol, the stress hormone, can indirectly contribute to pigmentation by increasing inflammation and oxidative stress, which can overstimulate melanocytes.

Melasma, often called chloasma during pregnancy, is commonly seen as symmetrical brown patches on the face. It is triggered by the surge in oestrogen and progesterone, which increases the skin's sensitivity to UV exposure and stimulates excess melanin production. Similarly, women in perimenopause may experience melasma as fluctuating hormone levels impact melanocyte regulation.

Hormonal pigmentation is also linked to the use of oral contraceptives and HRT. These treatments introduce synthetic hormones that can mimic the effects of natural oestrogen and progesterone, potentially triggering melasma or worsening existing pigmentation. Managing this type of pigmentation is particularly challenging, as it requires not only topical treatments but also addressing the underlying hormonal influences, making sun protection and hormonal balance critical.

CLIENT EDUCATION AND REALISTIC EXPECTATIONS

Pigmentation is a chronic condition and cannot simply be resolved with a one-off or a course of treatments. We continually produce new melanin in our skin and are exposed to the sun, making it crucial to maintain consistency in your treatment plans. You will need to continue using pigmentation-fighting ingredients in your skincare long-term to ensure that tyrosinase remains inhibited and pigmentation is kept at bay. The journey can take many months, but it is essential not to lose hope and change treatment mid-way through or mix up your skincare too quickly because you cannot see immediate results. It's also important to have realistic expectations; we are aiming to brighten the pigment, not achieve perfection. Throughout treatment, we continue to avoid pigmentation triggers, such as heat and sun, even in the maintenance phase, as this will reduce pigment production.

6

Laser Treatments & Skin Rejuvenation

INTRODUCTION TO ENERGY-BASED DEVICES

A laser is a powerful tool in a dermatology and skin clinic that can achieve so many excellent results. What is a laser? It's an instrument that generates a beam of light of a single wavelength that is collimated (parallel) and coherent (delivered in phase). Laser and light therapies are targeted treatments that utilise the benefits of focused light and energy sources to stimulate a wound healing response by targeting chromophores in the skin. Laser is a great non-surgical option for skin rejuvenation treatment. It can be utilised to target pigmentation, fine lines, irregular skin texture, vascular and unwanted hair growth. They are safe and effective, backed by evidence-based studies that provide excellent results when utilised correctly by a trained professional. This is a great way to help support skin health and can be a good little confidence boost.

HOW LIGHT AND LASER WORK

Laser and light-based therapies have become a cornerstone of modern skin rejuvenation, offering precise and effective solutions for concerns like pigmentation, redness, scarring, and aging. These treatments work by delivering controlled wavelengths of light or heat to specific targets in the skin, known as chromophores. Chromophores include pigment (melanin), blood vessels (hemoglobin), and even water in the skin. By selecting the right wavelength, energy is absorbed by the chromophore while leaving the surrounding tissue unharmed, stimulating repair and renewal.

LASER, IPL, AND LED – WHAT'S THE DIFFERENCE?

Laser: A laser emits a single, concentrated wavelength of light, allowing it to target a specific chromophore with high precision. For example, a pigment-specific laser can break down dark spots, while a vascular laser can close off broken capillaries. Because of their accuracy and power, lasers are ideal for treating distinct issues like pigmentation, tattoo removal, or deep resurfacing.

IPL (Intense Pulsed Light): Unlike lasers, IPL uses a broad spectrum of light that can target multiple chromophores simultaneously. By using filters, IPL can treat a range of issues such as redness, sun damage, and uneven skin tone in a single session. It's often used for full-face rejuvenation, as it can address both pigment and vascular concerns in one treatment.

LED (Light Emitting Diode): LED therapy is gentle and non-invasive, using low-level, therapeutic wavelengths to stimulate the skin's natural healing processes. LED treatments are painless and safe for all skin types, making them ideal for maintenance and recovery.

PHOTOTHERMAL AND PHOTOACOUSTIC EFFECTS

Two key mechanisms drive these treatments:
- **Photothermal effect:** Light energy is absorbed and converted into heat, which can destroy unwanted pigment cells, coagulate blood vessels, or stimulate collagen remodelling.
- **Photoacoustic effect:** Short pulses of light create a gentle shockwave that shatters pigment particles or ink in tattoos without harming surrounding tissue.

By combining these scientific principles, laser and light treatments can achieve impressive results with minimal downtime. Whether used for resurfacing, reducing pigmentation, calming redness, or boosting overall skin health, they offer a highly customizable approach that works at both the surface and deep structural levels of the skin.

COMMONLY TREATED CONCERNS:

- Pigmentation (sun damage, melasma, freckles)
- Vascular lesions (broken capillaries, rosacea, redness)
- Acne and acne scarring
- Skin texture and pores
- Fine lines and wrinkles
- Skin laxity and collagen loss
- Uneven skin tone or dullness

TYPES OF LASER AND LIGHT THERAPIES

Laser and light technologies have revolutionised modern skin treatments, offering solutions for redness, pigmentation, acne, aging, and overall skin rejuvenation. Each technology, IPL, LED, and various laser types, works in unique ways to target specific concerns with minimal damage to surrounding tissues.

IPL (Intense Pulsed Light)

IPL, often called "photo-rejuvenation," uses broad-spectrum light to target multiple chromophores, including pigment (melanin) and hemoglobin (in blood vessels). This makes it ideal for reducing redness, broken capillaries, sunspots, and uneven skin tone. Unlike a single-wavelength laser, IPL uses filters to adapt the light energy for different concerns, making it a versatile option for brightening and evening the complexion. With minimal downtime, IPL is perfect for those seeking a refreshed look without the recovery associated with more intensive treatments.

LED Light Therapy

LED therapy is a gentle, non-invasive treatment that uses specific wavelengths of light to stimulate natural skin functions:

- **Blue light:** Kills acne-causing bacteria, reducing active breakouts.
- **Red light:** Boosts collagen production, reduces inflammation, and accelerates healing.
- **Near-infrared light:** Penetrates deeply to promote cellular repair and tissue recovery.

LED is completely safe for all skin tones and types, with no downtime, making it a popular maintenance treatment to enhance overall skin health.

Ablative vs. Non-Ablative Lasers

Laser treatments can be classified into **ablative** and **non-ablative** categories:

- **Ablative lasers** (e.g., CO_2, Er: YAG) remove the outer layer of skin to resurface texture, reduce wrinkles, and erase deeper pigmentation. Results are dramatic but require downtime for healing.

- **Non-ablative lasers** (e.g., Nd: YAG, fractional lasers) heat deeper layers of the skin without removing the surface, stimulating collagen and tightening over time. These offer less downtime and gradual improvement.

Fractional Laser Resurfacing

Fractional lasers create micro-channels in the skin, triggering the body's natural healing response and boosting collagen remodelling. Because only a fraction of the skin is treated at a time, recovery is faster than with traditional ablative lasers. This makes fractional resurfacing a powerful option for improving fine lines, acne scarring, uneven texture, and deeper wrinkles while maintaining shorter healing periods.

BENEFITS OF LASER AND LIGHT TREATMENTS

Laser and light-based treatments offer robust, targeted solutions for a variety of skin concerns by working beneath the surface to stimulate natural healing and renewal processes. These treatments can significantly improve skin tone and clarity by reducing pigmentation, redness, and sun damage, resulting in a more even and radiant complexion. They also enhance skin texture by boosting collagen and elastin production, which helps to smooth fine lines, refine pores, and restore firmness over time. For those struggling with acne or scarring, specific laser modalities can target overactive oil glands, kill acne-causing bacteria, and remodel scar tissue for a more refined appearance. Beyond immediate results, laser treatments provide long-term skin health benefits, as the collagen stimulation and cellular turnover they initiate continue to improve the skin's structure and resilience for months after each session.

WHAT TO EXPECT DURING TREATMENT

Before any light-based therapies, you will have an in-depth consultation with your therapist, who will assess whether you are a safe and suitable candidate for treatment. They will assess your medical history, any current medications you are taking, previous reactions or responses to other treatments or allergens, goals and concerns.

It is recommended that a patch test be completed of the desired area in a small, discreet location to accurately assess how the skin will respond to the specific device and wavelengths chosen. This tool can help avoid undesirable outcomes and keep the patient safe.

During the appointment, while receiving the treatment, it can be normal to experience heat, zapping, tingling and a pain sensation. However, these sensations should only last while you are getting the treatment and should resolve shortly afterwards.

AFTERCARE AND DOWNTIME

After your treatment, you may experience some redness, sensitivity and mild swelling in the area. It is essential to avoid heat-inducing therapies, such as saunas or exercise, post-treatment, as this can prolong heat duration in the skin, which can, in turn, increase the length of downtime and prolong wound healing. Sun protection is crucial because you do not want to risk burning this sensitive area post-laser, as this can increase the risk of developing pigmentation. Soothing products are recommended in the days following laser as they can have a relaxing and cooling effect. Your technician may recommend an aftercare product that you can apply, which may contain ingredients like aloe vera to calm and soothe. This product is also light and non-occlusive, ensuring we don't trap heat within the skin.

RISKS AND SAFETY CONSIDERATIONS

It is always essential to have an in-depth consultation before consenting to any dermal treatment, but it is critical for laser and light-based therapies. It is necessary to have an in-depth consultation before reducing the possibility of side effects, as many can be reduced by following correct assessment, preparation, treatment and post-care protocols.

Mild side effects may include redness at the treated site, swelling and pigment changes. It is common for pigmentation to darken initially after treatment, but this should fade within days to weeks post-laser.

Less common side effects that are more serious may include: burns, scarring, and post-inflammatory hyperpigmentation (especially in darker skin tones). These side effects can be very distressing, potentially worsening the treated areas. Recognising this should underscore the importance of thorough laser preparation, consulting a qualified and experienced professional for these treatments, conducting a patch test, and adhering to the recommended aftercare. It is also essential to ensure the treatment will be completed with a TGA-approved device in clinical settings. Devices that have not been TGA-approved may be at heightened risk of adverse results as they are not appropriately regulated in Australia.

WHO IS A SUITABLE CANDIDATE?

Unfortunately, not everyone is a suitable candidate for laser treatments, and this isn't to be mean; it's to keep people safe. So, if a dermal therapist, doctor or nurse tells you that you aren't suitable for the treatment, this is simply because it is unsafe. You are at a higher risk of experiencing unwanted side effects such as burns and hyperpigmentation post-treatment.

Your laser technician will complete an in-depth assessment

before any treatment, and it may include questions such as your heritage and current medications. We may ask about your heritage and assess your skin colour against the Fitzpatrick scale, as darker Fitzpatrick individuals will be at a higher risk of burns than individuals with a lower Fitzpatrick scale. The medications that you are currently taking are also essential to check before EVERY appointment (as this can change frequently). Some medicines can make us photosensitive. This means that some medications, such as certain antibiotics, can increase your risk of burns and delayed wound healing, which could develop into PIHP. It is always important to discuss this with your technician before each treatment. We also do not recommend treatment to pregnant women.

It is also essential to be aware that it's unlikely that your concerns will be addressed entirely with only one treatment, so it is usual practice for your therapist to recommend a course of treatments that can take several months to complete before you reach your goal.

LONG-TERM SKIN MAINTENANCE

Laser is not a one-time treatment and often requires a course to treat the area thoroughly and may even require long-term annual or biannual therapies to keep it at bay over the long term. It is essential to develop an individualised skin plan with your skin therapist that is targeted to your concerns, that uses multiple modalities to keep your skin in check and feeling its best. This may include tyrosinase-inhibiting ingredients in our skincare, regular chemical exfoliating treatments, antioxidant powerhouse products to keep our skin resilient, and, of course, protecting our skin with SPF.

The sequence in which you complete your skin treatments will significantly improve your results and overall outcome. Before commencing any light-based treatment, it is essential to slowly prepare the skin so it can bounce back from the treatment quickly and safely. Rushing into high-intensity treatments too early can increase possible risks and side effects. Your practitioner may recommend that you start with small doses of active ingredients for 2-4 weeks before undergoing an in-clinic treatment. This will give your skin more resilience when it comes to in-clinic treatments. Then you will likely start with a mild skin preparation treatment such as a lactic peel. This gently exfoliates the skin, encouraging cell turnover, and allows the clinician to monitor how your skin responds to a low-level treatment before increasing the strength. It may be recommended to have a few peels before progressing to a laser treatment, depending on your skin type and its reaction to these treatments.

Consistency is key. Small changes done consistently over a long period of time give us the best benefits, so after a laser treatment, it's not the time to start skimping on your skincare routine!

7

Natural Skin Remedies: PRP, PDO threads

WHAT IS BIO-STIMULATION?

This process involves a skin treatment that encourages the body to produce its own collagen and elastin. This can be achieved through various modalities, including skin treatments like chemical peels and skin needling. However, we observe more significant improvements when using injectable biostimulators, such as PRP and PDO threads. This is ideal for clients looking to improve their skin quality, restore volume loss, and achieve skin tightening. This is an excellent alternative for individuals who are not interested in adding volume through the means of injectable treatments. These treatments offer numerous benefits, including tightening loose skin, enhancing skin luminosity and clarity, brightening dark circles, and boosting collagen and elastin to thicken crepey skin. Although these treatments can yield excellent results, it's essential to understand that they involve causing trauma to the skin and allowing it to heal. Consequently, results take time, and this is not a quick fix. Your skin is often considered a journey, and taking the natural route will take time (think months to a year), but trust me, investing in your skin is never a waste.

UNDERSTANDING COLLAGEN AND AGING

Collagen is the most abundant protein in the skin, providing firmness and structure. From the age of 25, our collagen and elastin supplies start to decline, which is why we notice signs of ageing. Loss of our collagen can result in thinning skin, fine lines and sagging skin. Through methods of bio stimulation, you can boost collagen and elastin production again, which can restore the skin's quality.

WHAT ARE THREAD LIFTS?

This is a hot topic that many people are very intrigued by, and I often receive questions about it. This is a great way to lift sagging tissues when the addition of more volume is not the primary concern. Thread lifts are often barbed threads of Polydioxanone (which is the same material that surgical dissolvable sutures are made from). This product blends with the skin without irritating, yet is strong enough to lift and hold tissues for months. These threads stay in the skin and dissolve over 6 months, but during the initial few months, they stimulate the growth of new collagen and elastin surrounding the threads to lift and improve the quality of the surrounding skin. This can add to a more lifted and enhanced appearance.

TYPES OF THREADS AND THEIR FUNCTIONS

When we mention threads, we're referring to several types that operate differently to achieve slightly different results.

Mono threads: fine, smooth threads placed into the skin to improve skin quality. These fine dissolvable sutures are inserted into the skin with a needle in large quantities to promote an inflammatory response in the skin, which can, in turn, stimulate the production of collagen and elastin. This helps support and grow healthy new skin in the treated area, which can produce smoother and thicker skin. After these threads are placed, it is normal not to see any results for the first 6-8 weeks. But from that time, results can gradually improve over the coming months.

Screw threads: used for areas needing volume stimulation (e.g., nasolabial folds). They work in a similar way to mono threads, but they are spiralised around the needle, which can provide more lift and definition in the treated area. This is a great option to use in deep lines or folds such as the nasolabial folds. After these threads are placed, it is normal not to see any results for the first 6-8 weeks.

Cog or barbed threads: Most threads provide mechanical lift and anchoring in areas like the jawline or cheeks. They use 4-8 barbed threads placed near the hairline, down along the jaw, cheeks, midface, neck and brows to offer an instant lift result. Although these threads seem to give instant results, that's not without risks, and a thorough consultation with a qualified practitioner is required before consenting to treatment.

It is also common practice and beneficial to use these threads in combination with each other to treat various areas. Cog threads can be used to lift the mid face, neck and brows. Mono threads can be used to treat crepey skin in the neck, as well as accordion lines, perioral lines, and around the eyes. And screw threads can be placed in nasolabial folds and deep accordion lines to achieve more lift.

WHAT TO EXPECT DURING A THREAD TREATMENT

This is an in-clinic treatment, so a thorough analysis and consultation are completed, and the client will receive their bespoke treatment plan. If they are deemed a suitable candidate for this procedure, they are given time to consider the treatment, ensuring they understand the procedure and are happy to proceed. Once they have decided, they can book their preferred treatment date. I always recommend this be booked just before having some time off, such as a long weekend or holiday (although they are unable to fly for the weeks following the treatment).

The procedure is completed in the clinic in around 45 minutes to 1.5 hours under local anaesthetic. The threads are inserted with a cannula or a needle into the treatment area. Once numb, it is common for the client to experience a tugging sensation; however, if numbed effectively, it should not be too uncomfortable. It is normal to experience swelling and possible bruising post this treatment. Cog threads are going to provide an immediate lifting effect (although keep in mind this result is likely to drop a bit over the 2 weeks following the treatment). All types of threads (mono, screw, and cog) will take around 6-12 weeks to produce boosted collagen and elastin, so unfortunately, it is a slow process.

HOW THREADS WORK OVERTIME

When PDO threads are inserted into the skin, the body identifies them as a biocompatible foreign object, triggering a controlled wound-healing cascade. This process begins at the cellular level with the activation of immune cells, particularly macrophages and neutrophils, which release cytokines and growth factors such as TGF-β (Transforming Growth Factor Beta) and PDGF (Platelet-Derived Growth Factor). These biochemical messengers recruit and activate fibroblasts, the key architects of skin regeneration. Once activated, fibroblasts migrate to the area and begin synthesising the extracellular matrix (ECM), specifically collagen types I and III, elastin, and hyaluronic acid. Collagen provides structural integrity, elastin allows the skin to stretch and bounce back, and hyaluronic acid retains moisture, together forming the "holy trinity" of youthful, resilient skin.

Simultaneously, the threads initiate neovascularisation, or new blood vessel formation, through upregulation of VEGF (Vascular Endothelial Growth Factor). This improves microcirculation, enhancing oxygen and nutrient delivery to the dermal tissue, which accelerates cell metabolism and supports long-term skin health. Over several weeks to months, this microenvironment becomes richer, denser, and more functional, with increased dermal thickness, improved hydration, and visibly enhanced texture and elasticity.

Unlike treatments that merely plump or paralyse, PDO threads work by bio-stimulating the skin's natural healing intelligence. As the threads slowly dissolve, they leave behind a scaffold of newly deposited collagen fibres, continuing to support the skin long after the material itself is gone. It's this elegant, cell-driven repair process that gives thread lifting its reputation for natural-looking, progressive rejuvenation not by altering facial anatomy, but by revitalising it from within.

OTHER BIO-STIMULATING TREATMENTS

Polynucleotides (PN/PNH/PRP): stimulate regeneration, hydration, and repair with the use of Salmon DNA. This can improve the quality, texture, and clarity of the skin.

Poly-L-lactic acid: collagen stimulator for gradual volume replenishment. This treatment triggers an inflammatory response in the skin, prompting it to produce its own collagen and elastin around the poly-l-lactic acid threads of boluses.

Skin boosters: hydrate and support collagen from within. This is an excellent hyaluronic acid, often containing added vitamins and minerals, which is injected superficially all over the skin to boost the skin's hydration levels and stimulate collagen and elastin.

Micro needling with growth factors triggers a healing cascade to improve skin quality, clarity, texture, and lumosity. This is achieved through standard micro-needling, combined with the topical application of growth factors that penetrate deeper into the skin by sliding into the newly created channels.

IDEAL CANDIDATES FOR THREADS AND BIO-STIMULATORS

Clients who are often most suitable for biostimulators have mild to moderate skin laxity. If the skin is too loose, they may not have effective results from these treatments. They may have early signs of jowling or volume loss that can be addressed with some skin-improving treatments. They often desire subtle rejuvenation without drastic change and want to improve the overall health of their skin, but their skin is not too weathered or at a stage of requiring surgical intervention. The healthcare professional will assess whether a candidate is unsuitable for treatment. Common reasons may include poor wound healing due to diabetes or autoimmune conditions, active infections or acne at the site, pregnancy or breastfeeding, or the client's poor physical condition. There are additional criteria where a client may not be suitable for treatment at that time, but this is assessed on a case-by-case basis.

RISKS AND CONSIDERATIONS

As with any treatment, this procedure does not come without risks. These should be discussed with your health professional before having any treatment. But some of the risks include:

- Swelling (mild to moderate)

- Bruising
- Asymmetry (usually temporary)

Rare risks may include:
- Thread extrusion
- Infection
- Puckering

It's essential to choose a qualified, experienced professional when considering PDO thread treatments. These procedures require not only a skilled injector, but also strict adherence to sterile technique to minimise the risk of infection or complications. PDO threads are TGA-approved medical devices, and as such, they must be administered in a clinical setting by a trained practitioner. A proper consultation, thorough assessment, and informed consent are crucial to ensure both safety and personalised results.

LONGEVITY AND MAINTENANCE

Mono threads: Results take 6-8 weeks to start working and continue to improve over the following months. It is recommended that the treatment be repeated every 6–12 months for optimal skin quality and improvement.

Lifting threads: results can last 12–24 months, depending on the product and individual response. Results are immediate, but it's normal for the threads to drop and settle within the first two weeks.

Maintenance may include combining with LED, peels, skin needling and lasers. A qualified professional should make a personalised treatment plan.

Biostimulators are a great option to improve the quality and appearance of your skin without adding any extra volume or changing the way that you look. This is a great alternative and/or addition to other cosmetic aesthetic treatments that are available. This can create a subtle enhancement and support the long-term health of the skin.

8

Skincare Products: What Really Works?

WHY SKINCARE MATTERS

Our skin is our body's largest organ and its first line of defence against environmental stressors like UV rays, pollution, and bacteria. A consistent, bespoke skincare routine helps maintain the skin's barrier, supports cell renewal, and keeps the complexion looking vibrant and healthy. Our skin is the only one we'll ever have, so it deserves consistent care because when we look after it, it will continue to protect and serve us well into our later years. Skincare is also the basis for how your skin looks and can influence and improve the effects of your in-clinic treatments. You will often hear skin specialists say that your home routine accounts for 90% of your results, and this can be very true!

UNDERSTANDING YOUR SKIN TYPE

Before choosing products, it's essential to identify your skin type, as this guides what ingredients and textures will work best. Common skin types include:

- **Normal:** Balanced, neither too oily nor dry
- **Oily:** Excess sebum production, prone to shine and breakouts
- **Dry:** Lacking moisture, may feel tight or flaky
- **Combination:** Oily in some areas (usually T-zone), dry or normal elsewhere
- **Sensitive:** Easily irritated or reactive to products and environmental factors

THE SKIN BARRIER AND WHY IT'S VITAL

The skin barrier is a protective layer made of lipids and cells that retains moisture and blocks harmful agents. Damage to this barrier leads to dryness, sensitivity, redness, and accelerated aging. Essential skincare supports and repairs the barrier daily. As discussed earlier, it's important to look after the microbiome of our skin to ensure that our barrier is functioning to the best of its ability. Once this becomes unbalanced, it can take a long time to bring it back to health. Prevention is always more effective than cure.

THE BASICS: YOUR DAILY SKINCARE ROUTINE

It's essential to get the basics down pat before we start expanding our routine to include various serums and active ingredients. I always ensure that my clients have at least a cleanser, moisturiser, and SPF, and use these products for a few weeks to ensure their skin has a positive response to the products before increasing the frequency. I believe it's best to proceed with caution and introduce new skincare products slowly to minimise the disruption to your barrier. Take some time to adapt to changes; I find that making minor adjustments over a few months has the least adverse effects.

A simple, consistent routine is best for all skin types. The core steps are:

- **Cleansing:** Removes dirt, oil, and makeup without stripping natural oils. The type of cleanser you use will be dependent on your skin type.
- **Moisturising:** Hydrates and locks in moisture to keep skin soft and hydrated
- **Sun Protection:** Shields skin from harmful UVA and UVB rays to prevent premature aging and skin cancer

CLEANSERS: CHOOSING THE RIGHT ONE

There are various types of face washes, making it difficult to determine which one is best suited for your skin type and needs. When considering options like a gel, foam, cream, balm, or oil, how can you choose between them? First, it is essential to decipher what type of skin you have. If you have oily skin, a gel or foam may be a better choice for you. If you have dry and irritated skin, a non-irritating cream cleanser may be a better option for you. Below, I have highlighted the different types of cleansers available and how to choose the right one for you.

Cream cleanser: A gentle, hydrating cleanser designed to nourish and restore dry, dehydrated, and/or damaged skin types, without stripping the skin or disrupting the micro-biome balance. Often opaque in colour, non foaming and can leave a little residue on the skin to increase hydration.

Gel cleanser: A deeply cleansing wash that often turns to a foam for improving the lather. This can be great for removing thick layers of makeup, dirt, and impurities from the skin and usually contains an acid such as lactic, glycolic, or salicylic for improved cleansing and resurfacing effects. This product is ideal for oily and mature skin types, but it's not recommended for individuals with impaired skin barriers, as it may cause stripping.

Oil cleanser: An oil-based cleanser that helps to dissolve stubborn sebum, sunscreen and makeup. They are popular with double cleansing routines to remove the initial buildup, followed by a gel or foaming cleanser to cleanse the pores deeply. They are great for dry to standard skin types but can also be beneficial for oily skin if used as part of a double cleanse method.

Foaming cleanser: A light and airy cleanser that helps to lift away oil and impurities. This is an excellent choice for oily, acne-prone skin. They provide a deep clean and don't require too much pressure or rubbing, which can be beneficial with painful acne lesions, but can be stripping to the skin, so it is not suitable for impaired barriers.

Balm cleanser: A solid, oil-based cleanser in a thick balm form that turns into an oil when heated in the balms before application. Great for removing oil, impurities and makeup, then when water is applied, it emulsifies into a light milky form. Suitable for all skin types and effective in the first cleanse of a double cleanse routine.

Powder cleansers: Great for a deep exfoliation and refresh of the skin. It is often not recommended to use them daily, as they may strip the skin. This cleanser comes as a powder that is tipped into the hand and mixed with a few drops of water to create an exfoliating paste used to cleanse the skin. Usually, it is recommended to be used 1-2x weekly and is more beneficial for oily skin types.

Micellar water/ makeup wipes: Great for removing stubborn eye makeup without irritating delicate areas. Although it is not considered an effective cleanse after wearing makeup. It is essential to follow up with a deep cleanse after using a makeup wipe. It is also necessary to know that many of these products contain fragrances that may irritate delicate or impaired skin types.

Whichever cleanser you choose for your skin, it is essential to ensure that it accommodates your individual skin type and is pH-balanced to ensure that it doesn't disrupt your skin barrier. Be sure to avoid harsh products containing strong fragrances, as this is a common cause of an irritated skin barrier.

MOISTURISERS: HYDRATION AND BARRIER SUPPORT

Choosing the right moisturiser for you is like choosing your cleanser. Different skin types will also tolerate moisturisers differently. Someone with oily, acne-prone skin is going to prefer a lightweight, oil-free option, as this will not aggravate sebum production or cause unnecessary inflammation in the skin. For someone with dehydrated skin, a rich, thick, hydrating cream is ideal, as it provides an instant cooling and hydrating sensation, eliminating the uncomfortable tightness and/or stinging sensation. Moisturiser is an essential step in the skincare routine after cleansing, as it replaces the skin's hydration, reduces irritation, and enhances the effectiveness of other treatments.

The different types of moisturisers are:

Humectants, Such as glycerine and hyaluronic acid (HA), are effective at attracting moisture to the skin through the air and encourage water retention in the skin. Ideal for dehydrated skin types that require additional hydration.

Emollients: Such as ceramides and lanolin. Soften and smooth the skin. Offer rich hydration and often contain mineral oils.

Occlusives: A thick paste moisturiser often made with beeswax or petroleum, which creates an effective protective barrier to prevent moisture loss in the skin. This is common with "slugging" techniques and with impaired skin barriers. Although these moisturisers can sometimes feel heavy on the skin, not everyone will tolerate them well. In acne-prone skin, they can cause breakouts.

SUN PROTECTION: YOUR MOST IMPORTANT STEP

Sunscreen is your skin's best defence against pigmentation, ageing, and skin cancer. UVA rays penetrate windows and reach deep into the skin, causing ageing and worsening pigmentation, even in the shade. UVB causes sunburn and direct DNA damage, leading to skin cancer. Apply **one teaspoon to the face** and reapply every **4 hours** (more if sweating or swimming). Mineral (physical) sunscreens are best for pigmentation as they reflect UV and don't create heat like chemical sunscreens. Choose **SPF 50+** for reliable protection. Sunscreen is your most effective anti-ageing and pigmentation-fighting tool — wear it daily, no excuses!

TARGETED TREATMENTS: WHEN AND HOW TO INTRODUCE THEM

Antioxidants: Antioxidants in skincare help protect your skin from free radical damage caused by UV rays, pollution, and stress, which can lead to premature ageing and pigmentation. They work by neutralising these unstable molecules before they cause damage to collagen, elastin, and skin cells. Ingredients like Vitamin C, Vitamin E, niacinamide, and green tea are potent antioxidants that brighten skin, improve texture, and reduce inflammation. Adding antioxidants to your routine is as simple as using a serum in the morning before sunscreen for extra protection. Consistent daily use helps strengthen your skin's barrier and keeps it looking youthful, radiant, and healthy.

Chemical exfoliants (AHAs, BHAs) promote cell turnover and are great for brightening and tightening our skin. It should be introduced gradually to prevent skin irritation. We want these acids to exfoliate our skin gently; more is not always better.

Retinoids (also known as vitamin A): Help by improving texture and stimulating the production of collagen. However, it may irritate if overused or introduced at too high a strength for your skin to adjust to. This is best under professional guidance so that you can contact them for protocols and advice.

It is always important to patch test new products to prevent a reaction once it has been applied all over. Active ingredients are strong, which is great because they can get you excellent results, but it's essential to proceed with caution. Begin with one or two sessions per week for a few weeks. If you don't experience any reaction, increase to 3-4 sessions per week. After approximately two months, you should be able to use it daily. If you experience redness, irritation, or stinging at this time, it may be too much and is best to reduce the use or discontinue completely until your skin returns to normal. Then reintroduce again slowly once settled.

AVOIDING COMMON SKINCARE MISTAKES

Over-cleansing: <u>Take the time to work out which cleanser is right for you.</u> Be gentle with your skin, we are trying to clean it, not traumatise it. Use your hands, a gentle cleansing device or a clean towel. We prefer to avoid harsh scrubbing devices as they may cause microtears in your skin and could affect the balance of your microbiome.

Using too many actives: Always prioritise your primary skin concern first, and gradually introduce active ingredients to avoid disrupting your skin's natural balance or compromising the skin barrier.   It is recommended to incorporate active ingredients slowly, e.g., 1-2x weekly for a month, then increase to 3-4x weekly for another month before using daily. Use a product for at least a month before adding more actives, allowing your skin plenty of time to adjust. If you notice signs of irritation, discontinue using the products until your skin tolerates them well and can proceed.

Skipping sunscreen: As discussed earlier, sunscreen is essential in your skincare to protect you from sun damage, but more importantly when you are using actives in your skincare. This is due to their exfoliating properties, which may resurface the top layer of your skin, making you more susceptible to damage and ageing. Therefore, protection of this fresh skin is essential. Otherwise, it can make ageing and pigmentation worse!

Changing products too frequently: Remember, our skin takes at least 30 days to turn over. It's normal not to see immediate changes or results from a vitamin C or vitamin

A product. Try the product for at least 2 months before considering a change, as this allows your skin to show whether it will be effective or not. Keep in mind that this is different from reacting to a product, which should be discontinued. And when it comes to depigmentation treatments and products, the process of formation and removal may take even longer.

PROFESSIONAL SKINCARE: WHEN TO SEEK HELP

When you are experiencing persistent concerns like acne, pigmentation, rosacea, or eczema, it is essential to understand that you may not be able to cure all of your problems by yourself and may need the assistance of a professional. They can provide an in-depth consultation and skin analysis, create a bespoke treatment plan and provide effective treatments to get your skin back into peak health as soon as possible. They also participate in regular science-based training, so they can tell you if the video you saw on TikTok last week is real or fake news. As you will be on a treatment plan, you will attend the clinic monthly, or sometimes more regularly, allowing them to check in with you regularly to see what is working and what isn't, so that it can be changed accordingly. These regular check-ins are essential to prevent barrier disturbance or incorrect products/treatments, which may create further problems for you.

LIFESTYLE FACTORS THAT AFFECT SKIN HEALTH

Hydration: Drink plenty of water daily; around 2L is generally ideal for healthy body functioning. You will notice that when you are dehydrated, your skin is also dehydrated.

Nutrition: A Balanced diet rich in antioxidants, vitamins, and healthy fats is essential for healthy skin. The overconsumption of saturated fats, sugar, carbohydrates, and dairy can all add to inflammation and an overproduction of oil in your skin.

Sleep: When we sleep at night, our body heals and regenerate themselves. Quality REM sleep supports healthy skin repair.

Stress management and avoiding smoking play key roles in keeping your skin healthy. Stress and smoking create inflammation in our body and interfere with skin healing processes, making our skin more prone to damage and ageing.

SKINCARE IS A JOURNEY

Consistency and patience are key. Most improvements take weeks to months. Remember, our skin takes at least 30 days to turn over, and this slows down further as we age. So sometimes things can take longer than we like but stick with it and you just might be surprised!

Build your routine slowly to ensure long-term success and commitment. I always like to start simple with a cleanser, moisturiser, and SPF, then slowly add products to target your concerns over the course of a few months. This will allow the skin to adjust to the changes in routine slowly, making it easier for you to form this new habit and avoid feeling overwhelmed.

Also, keep in mind that everyone's skin is unique. Just because a skincare product or routine works well for your friend doesn't mean it will work well for you. Personalise your routine to suit your needs, lifestyle, and preferences. If you are stuck, I strongly recommend consulting a professional for an in-depth consultation and skin examination to ensure your skin receives the best care from day one.

9

Holistic Skincare — The Role of Lifestyle, Stress & Sleep

Our skin is often the first to reveal what's going on inside our bodies. Late nights show up as dark circles. Stress can manifest as breakouts, redness, or flare-ups. A poor diet can leave skin looking dull, while glowing, clear skin is almost always the result of balanced internal health. This is because our skin is not an isolated organ; it's a dynamic reflection of our internal systems, from hormones to gut health to our mental and emotional well-being.

The modern beauty industry tends to focus on topical products and quick fixes, promising radiant results in a matter of days. While these solutions can certainly help, true skin transformation happens when you look beyond the surface. Holistic skincare is about addressing the root cause of skin concerns, balancing the body from within, supporting cellular health, and nurturing mental wellness. So, your glow is sustainable and authentic.

In this chapter, we'll explore how stress, sleep, diet, supplements, gut health, and daily habits shape your skin's appearance and resilience. You'll learn why chronic stress leads to inflammation and early aging, why sleep is the ultimate skin treatment, and how simple changes in your daily routine can make a profound difference to your complexion.

What Does "Holistic Skincare" Actually Mean?

Holistic skincare is a shift in mindset. It's about moving from a reactive approach (covering up or "fixing" problems) to a proactive one and creating a lifestyle that naturally prevents skin concerns before they arise.

- **Nutrition as a foundation:** Your skin cells are made from the nutrients you consume. Without sufficient vitamins, minerals, and healthy fats, the skin struggles to repair itself, leading to premature aging, dryness, and breakouts.
- **Hormonal balance:** Fluctuations in estrogen, progesterone, and testosterone can cause acne, pigmentation, or sensitivity. Holistic skincare works with the body to maintain hormonal harmony through stress management, balanced eating, and movement.
- **Detoxification:** The liver, lymphatic system, and kidneys are your body's detox powerhouses. When these systems are overloaded (due to poor diet, alcohol, or stress), the skin often becomes a

secondary detox organ, resulting in blemishes or irritation.

- **Gut health:** A well-functioning gut absorbs nutrients efficiently and prevents inflammation that can surface on the skin.

Unlike conventional beauty routines that rely heavily on surface treatments, holistic skincare prioritises internal health and prevention. Think of it as creating fertile soil before planting a garden. If the foundation is strong, the results are vibrant and lasting.

GLOW FROM WITHIN: HOW INTERNAL WELLNESS SHAPES YOUR SKIN

Your skin is your body's largest organ, and its health reflects your overall wellness. Many common skin concerns are symptoms of imbalance, not just external issues. For example:

- A dull complexion might be linked to dehydration or lack of antioxidants.
- Red, inflamed patches can be a sign of stress, gut irritation, or food sensitivities.
- Premature fine lines and sagging often stem from chronic inflammation, oxidative stress, and lack of restorative sleep.

Holistic skincare encourages you to look beyond surface-level "fixes." Instead of asking, *What product will cover this problem? You ask, what is my skin trying to tell me?*

Example: A person with recurring hormonal acne might try countless cleansers and spot treatments with little success. But once they support their hormones with a lower-sugar diet, manage stress, and improve sleep, their skin clears significantly.

STRESS AND THE SKIN

Stress is one of the most common yet underestimated triggers for skin problems. When we're stressed, our bodies produce cortisol, often referred to as the "stress hormone." While short bursts of cortisol can help us stay alert in challenging situations, chronic stress keeps cortisol levels elevated, causing a cascade of skin issues:

1. **Increased Inflammation:** Cortisol amplifies inflammatory responses, worsening acne, eczema, rosacea, and psoriasis.
2. **Weakened Skin Barrier:** High cortisol reduces ceramide and lipid production, making the skin more prone to dryness, irritation, and redness.
3. **Pigmentation Flare-ups:** Cortisol can overstimulate melanocytes (pigment-producing cells), leading to stubborn dark patches or melasma.
4. **Delayed Healing:** Elevated stress slows cell turnover,

meaning blemishes, wounds, or post-treatment healing take longer.

DAILY STRESS-RELIEF PRACTICES FOR HEALTHY SKIN

- **Mindful Breathing:** Just 3–5 minutes of deep, controlled breathing can lower cortisol and shift your body into a state of calm.
- **Movement:** Yoga, Pilates, walking, or dancing are all effective at reducing stress hormones and improving circulation (which delivers nutrients and oxygen to your skin).
- **Nature Time:** Spending even 15 minutes outdoors lowers cortisol and boosts mood.
- **Journaling or Meditation:** Writing out thoughts or practicing guided meditation can reduce emotional stress.

Tip: If your skin flares up after stressful periods (like exams or deadlines), consider incorporating adaptogenic herbs (such as ashwagandha or rhodiola) into your routine. These herbs help regulate cortisol levels and improve resilience, but always check with a healthcare provider first.

SLEEP: YOUR SKIN'S BEST TREATMENT

Sleep isn't just about rest—it's when your body goes into active repair mode. During the night, skin cells switch from protecting (which they do during the day) to healing and regeneration.

WHY SLEEP MATTERS FOR YOUR SKIN:

- **Boosts Collagen:** Deep sleep stimulates the release of growth hormone, which triggers collagen production for firmer, smoother skin.
- **Reduces Inflammation:** Poor sleep raises stress hormones, which inflame the skin and slow healing.
- **Prevents Puffiness and Dark Circles:** Lack of rest affects blood circulation and fluid retention, causing under-eye bags and dullness.
- **Enhances Product Absorption:** Overnight, skin permeability increases, meaning serums and moisturisers work more effectively while you sleep.

SLEEP HYGIENE FOR RADIANT SKIN:

- Stick to a consistent sleep schedule (even on weekends) to regulate your body's natural rhythm.
- Dim the lights and avoid screens at least an hour before bed—blue light interferes with melatonin

production, your sleep hormone.

- Use a silk pillowcase to reduce friction and prevent sleep creases.
- Apply a nourishing night cream or oil (with ceramides, peptides, or hyaluronic acid) to prevent overnight moisture loss.
- If you struggle to fall asleep, try natural aids like magnesium, warm herbal tea (chamomile, valerian), or calming scents like lavender.

GUT HEALTH & GLOWING SKIN

Your gut and your skin are deeply connected, a concept known as the **gut–skin axis**. An imbalanced gut micro-biome (too many harmful bacteria and not enough good ones) can trigger systemic inflammation that shows up on your skin.

SIGNS YOUR GUT MAY BE AFFECTING YOUR SKIN:

- Frequent bloating, constipation, or digestive dis-comfort.
- Acne or rosacea flare-ups after eating certain foods.
- Unexplained rashes, dullness, or stubborn conges-tion.

GUT-FRIENDLY FOODS FOR HEALTHY SKIN:

- **Prebiotics & Probiotics:** Foods like kimchi, sauerkraut, kefir, and yogurt help populate your gut with healthy bacteria.
- **Healthy Fats:** Omega-3-rich foods like salmon, flaxseed, and walnuts reduce inflammation and improve skin elasticity.
- **Antioxidants:** Leafy greens, berries, and colourful vegetables neutralise free radicals that cause premature aging.
- **Zinc & Vitamin A:** Found in pumpkin seeds, liver, and sweet potatoes—these nutrients support skin repair and regulate oil production.

Tip: Minimise processed foods, high-sugar snacks, and alcohol, which can disrupt gut flora and lead to flare-ups.

ALCOHOL, SUGAR & LIFESTYLE HABITS

Alcohol:

Alcohol dehydrates the body and skin, depleting vitamin A (essential for cell turnover). Regular drinking can cause redness, puffiness, and accelerate fine lines due to inflammation. If you do drink:

- Alternate each alcoholic drink with water.
- Choose lower-sugar options like dry wines or spirits with soda water.

- Rehydrate with electrolytes the next day.

Sugar:

High sugar intake leads to glycation, a process where sugar molecules bind to collagen and elastin, making them stiff and less elastic. This speeds up aging. To reduce glycation:

- Pair sweet treats with protein or fibre to stabilise blood sugar spikes.
- Swap refined sugar for natural sweeteners like stevia or small amounts of honey.

DAILY HABITS THAT MAKE A VISIBLE DIFFERENCE

1. **Hydration:** Aim for 2-3 litres of water daily. Add a pinch of sea salt or a squeeze of lemon to improve absorption.
2. **Facial Massage & Lymphatic Drainage:** Tools like gua sha or even your hands help move stagnant fluid, reduce puffiness, and boost circulation for a natural glow.
3. **Exercise:** Movement increases blood flow, delivering oxygen and nutrients to the skin while promoting detox through sweat.
4. **SPF:** Sun exposure is responsible for up to 80% of visible aging. Use a broad-spectrum SPF 50 daily, even on cloudy days or indoors (UV rays penetrate

windows).

5. **Supplements:** Zinc, omega-3 fatty acids, vitamin D, probiotics, and collagen peptides are great skin-supporting supplements. Always consult a healthcare professional for dosing.

6. **B12 and NAD+ Injections:** These injectable therapies are gaining popularity for energy, cellular repair, and skin tone improvements. B12 helps reduce fatigue and can improve circulation, while NAD+ supports mitochondrial health and may slow skin aging.

THE MIND-SKIN CONNECTION

Our emotional well-being directly affects our skin. Ever noticed how your face glows when you're happy or how a stressful week can lead to breakouts? This is because the skin and brain share close communication pathways.

- **Chronic anxiety or depression** can increase inflammation and oxidative stress and reduce your skin's ability to heal.
- **Mindfulness practices** like meditation, yoga, and gratitude journaling can help regulate nervous system responses, lowering inflammation and creating a calmer complexion.

YOUR HOLISTIC SKIN ACTION PLAN

To truly transform your skin from the inside out:

1. **Prioritise rest:** Aim for 7-9 hours of quality sleep each night.
2. **Reduce stress:** Create a daily 10-minute ritual-breathwork, meditation, or even a short walk.
3. **Eat a skin-friendly diet:** Focus on whole foods, healthy fats, and plenty of antioxidants.
4. **Stay hydrated:** Keep water nearby and drink consistently throughout the day.
5. **Protect your skin barrier:** Use gentle skincare, SPF, and avoid harsh, stripping products.
6. **Support your gut:** Include probiotic and prebiotic-rich foods and minimise alcohol and processed sugar.
7. **Be consistent:** Small daily habits add up to the most significant changes.

10

Hormones and Your Skin

Women's skin is a living reflection of internal rhythms - especially hormones. These chemical messengers constantly influence our skin's appearance, texture, and behaviour throughout the month. If you've ever wondered why your face looks radiant one week and oily or breakout-prone the next, hormones are often the reason.

The three key players —estrogen, progesterone, and testosterone — fluctuate in a cycle that repeats approximately every 28 days. Their rise and fall shape everything from oil production to collagen levels, water retention, and inflammation.

- **Estrogen:** Often referred to as the "glow hormone," estrogen helps maintain hydration, elasticity, and firmness by stimulating collagen, elastin, and hyaluronic acid production. When estrogen levels are high (especially in the follicular phase), skin appears plumper, smoother, and brighter.
- **Progesterone:** This hormone takes the lead in the

second half of the cycle (the luteal phase) and is known for increasing sebum production, which can lead to congestion, clogged pores, and breakouts in some women. It also contributes to water retention, which explains the puffiness or bloating many notice before their period.

- **Testosterone:** Although women produce much less testosterone than men, its effects are still powerful. Spikes around ovulation and the luteal phase can drive oil production, sometimes tipping the skin into overdrive and leading to acne flare-ups or a shiny T-zone.

These hormonal shifts influence oiliness, barrier strength, sensitivity, and inflammation - meaning your skin's needs aren't constant throughout the month. Learning to anticipate these changes and adapt your skincare accordingly can transform not only your skin but also your mindset. Rather than seeing your skin as unpredictable, you begin to view its fluctuations as part of a natural rhythm.

WHY HORMONES MATTER BEYOND APPEARANCE

Hormones do much more than affect how your skin looks - they determine how it functions:

- **Estrogen:** Encourages wound healing, boosts

antioxidant protection, and supports a healthy skin barrier. When estrogen drops (as it does during menstruation or in perimenopause), skin may become drier, more sensitive, and prone to redness.

- **Progesterone:** Known for its calming, nurturing qualities, it can also make the skin feel thicker or slightly swollen due to water retention, especially during the luteal phase.

- **Testosterone:** Stimulates sebaceous glands to produce oil. While a bit of oil is essential for healthy skin, excess can lead to clogged pores, blackheads, and inflammation if not balanced with proper cleansing and exfoliation.

Understanding these dynamics helps you stop fighting your skin's natural rhythms and start working with them, just as you would adapt your exercise or diet to match your energy levels during the month.

WEEK-BY-WEEK SKIN SHIFTS

Week 1: Menstruation (Days 1–7)

Your cycle starts with menstruation. Both estrogen and progesterone are at their lowest, and skin may feel dry, sensitive, or lacklustre. You might notice flare-ups of in-flammatory conditions like eczema or rosacea. Under-eye circles or puffiness are also common, thanks to fluid shifts and potential iron loss from bleeding.

What your skin needs:

- **Gentle hydration and barrier repair.** Use calming ingredients such as centella asiatica, panthenol, chamomile, or oat extract.
- **Avoid harsh actives** (like strong acids or retinoids) if your skin feels irritated or thin.
- **Lifestyle support:** Prioritise extra sleep and hydration to help your skin recover. Warm herbal teas (like nettle or raspberry leaf) can support circulation and reduce puffiness.

Week 2: Follicular Phase & Ovulation (Days 8–14)

As estrogen rises, your skin enters its **"golden week."** Skin looks clearer, smoother, and more radiant. Collagen production peaks, pores often appear smaller, and the texture is refined. This is the ideal time for treatments or introducing new active ingredients, as the skin barrier is at its strongest.

What your skin needs:

- **Brightening actives:** Vitamin C serums, alpha hydroxy acids (AHAs), and peptides work exceptionally well.
- **Professional treatments:** Consider scheduling facials, chemical peels, or skin needling for maximum results.

- **Lifestyle support:** You might feel more social and energised during this phase - hydrate well and consider increasing antioxidants in your diet (berries, leafy greens) to enhance your glow.

Week 3: Luteal Phase (Days 15–21)

Progesterone starts to climb, and testosterone may spike. This combination can increase oil production and lead to congestion, clogged pores, or breakouts - especially on the chin and jawline.

What your skin needs:

- **Clarifying and balancing ingredients:** Niacinamide, salicylic acid, zinc, or green tea can reduce oil and calm inflammation.
- **Spot treatments and clay masks:** These help keep pores clear and manage excess sebum.
- **Lifestyle support:** Reduce refined sugar and dairy, which can fuel inflammation and worsen breakouts. Adding magnesium and stress management (yoga, meditation) can help.

Week 4: Premenstrual (Days 22–28)

Inflammation is at its peak. Skin may feel sensitive, appear dull, or break out more. Puffiness and redness are also common, as is a general feeling of "heaviness" in the skin.

What your skin needs:

- **Anti-inflammatory care:** Aloe vera, green tea, chamomile, and ceramides are soothing choices.
- **Facial massage or gua sha:** These reduce puffiness by improving lymphatic drainage.
- **Avoid introducing new products:** Stick with nourishing, tried-and-true products to avoid irritation.

CYCLE-SYNCING YOUR SKINCARE

The idea of cycle-syncing your skincare means tailoring your routine to your body's needs during each phase:

- **Menstruation:** Hydration and calming ingredients. Gentle cleansers, rich moisturisers, and barrier support (like ceramides or squalane) work wonders.
- **Follicular Phase:** Focus on renewal and glow. Introduce exfoliants (AHAs, enzymes) and vitamin C. This is a good time for professional treatments or starting new products.
- **Luteal Phase:** Balance and detoxify. Use clarifying masks, anti-bacterial ingredients, and spot treatments.
- **Premenstrual:** Nourish and soothe. Think hydrating masks, calming oils (like jojoba or rosehip), and gentle massage.

Tip: Adjusting your routine slightly each week prevents overuse of actives, reduces irritation, and ensures your skin gets exactly what it needs when it needs it.

ACNE, PMS, & YOUR SKIN

Hormonal acne is a common premenstrual complaint. Driven by progesterone and testosterone, these breakouts often appear on the chin and jawline and can be cystic, painful, and slow to heal.

How to Manage Hormonal Acne:

- **Internal support:** Zinc, omega-3 fatty acids, and herbal aids like spearmint tea or chasteberry (Vitex) can reduce androgen activity.
- **Topical care:** Niacinamide, salicylic acid, and sulphur-based spot treatments can calm inflammation and clear bacteria.
- **LED therapy:** Blue light LED treatments are excellent for targeting acne-causing bacteria and reducing redness.

Mindset shift: Hormonal acne isn't a "failure." By tracking your cycle, you can anticipate these breakouts and start preventive measures (e.g., clay masks) before they appear.

CONTRACEPTIVES & HORMONAL DISRUPTION

Hormonal contraceptives (the pill, hormonal IUDs, implants) can significantly impact skin:

- **Oral contraceptive pill:** Often improves acne by reducing androgens, but can thin skin, increase pigmentation risk, and reduce hydration.
- **Post-pill acne:** When coming off the pill, hormones rebound, leading to flare-ups. Supporting the liver (cruciferous vegetables, lemon water), zinc, B vitamins, and adaptogens can ease this transition.
- **HRT (Hormone Replacement Therapy):** In menopause, HRT can improve skin thickness, hydration, and elasticity, though some women experience increased pigmentation or sensitivity.

Tip: Non-hormonal methods (like copper IUDs) don't directly affect hormones but still require observation, as other lifestyle shifts can change how your skin behaves.

HORMONE REPLACEMENT THERAPY (HRT) & SKIN HEALTH

During menopause, estrogen levels drop dramatically by as much as 30% in the first five years! This leads to thinner, drier skin, reduced collagen, slower wound healing, and a loss of elasticity. Hormone Replacement Therapy (HRT) can help counteract these effects by supplementing estrogen (and sometimes progesterone), restoring some of the skin's youthful resilience.

How HRT Benefits the Skin:

- **Boosts Collagen & Elasticity:** Estrogen stimulates fibroblast activity, increasing collagen and elastin for firmer, smoother skin.
- **Improves Hydration:** Estrogen enhances the skin's natural hyaluronic acid and lipid content, reducing dryness and flakiness.
- **Strengthens Barrier Function:** A healthier barrier means less irritation and greater protection from environmental damage.
- **Speeds Repair:** With improved cell turnover, post-treatment recovery and general healing are faster.

Potential Side Effects:

Some women experience pigmentation issues (melasma) due to estrogen's effect on melanocytes. Skin may also become temporarily sensitive to active ingredients like retinoids or AHAs. Rarely, an imbalance between estrogen and progesterone can trigger mild breakouts.

Skincare Tips on HRT:

- Wear broad-spectrum SPF 50 daily to counter pigmentation risks.

- Use hydrating and barrier-strengthening products with ceramides, hyaluronic acid, and squalene.
- Incorporate collagen-supporting ingredients like peptides and vitamin C.
- Choose a gentle exfoliation and monitor sensitivity when using actives.
- Address pigmentation with niacinamide, azelaic acid, or antioxidants.

Lifestyle Support:

Complement HRT with a diet rich in phytoestrogens (flaxseed, soy), omega-3 fatty acids, and antioxidants. Manage stress to prevent cortisol-related skin inflammation and consider collagen supplements to enhance firmness.

TRACKING & SKIN JOURNALING

Tracking your cycle and skin is one of the most empowering practices you can adopt. By noting how your skin looks and feels at different times of the month, you'll start to see patterns:

- Do you break out 3-5 days before your period?
- Is your skin radiant and clear mid-cycle?
- Do certain foods or stress levels make symptoms worse?

How to Track:

- Use apps like Flo, Clue, or MyFlo to track your cycle.
- Keep a skin journal - note breakouts, sensitivity, or changes in texture.
- Plan your skincare or treatments around your cycle. For example, book facials during your follicular phase for optimal results.

DIET & HORMONAL BALANCE

Your diet can either support or disrupt hormonal balance:

- Reduce inflammatory foods: Processed foods, refined sugars, and trans fats can worsen hormonal acne and inflammation.
- Eat hormone-supportive foods: Cruciferous vegetables (broccoli, cauliflower) help metabolise excess estrogen. Omega-3s (found in salmon and chia seeds) reduce inflammation and support hormone health.
- Stay hydrated: Hormonal shifts affect fluid retention; water and herbal teas help balance this.

STRESS & HORMONES

Stress increases cortisol, which in turn affects estrogen, progesterone, and testosterone balance. Chronic stress can lengthen PMS symptoms, worsen breakouts, and make the skin dull.

Stress reduction: Breathwork, journaling, and magnesium baths can all improve both mental state and skin clarity.

YOUR HORMONE-FRIENDLY SKIN ACTION PLAN

1. **Track your cycle** for 2–3 months to spot patterns.
2. **Adapt your skincare** each week (hydration → glow → balancing → soothing).
3. **Support your hormones internally** with diet, supplements, and rest.
4. **Book treatments strategically** (e.g., avoid harsh peels during PMS when skin is more reactive).
5. **Be kind to your skin**—fluctuations are normal and natural.

THE JOURNEY DOESN'T END AFTER TREATMENT

Cosmetic treatments are often seen as transformative milestones in our skin journey. The truth is that these treatments are not the final destination-they're a part of an ongoing relationship with your skin. The idea that a single procedure can "fix" everything is both misleading and limiting. Lasting results require more than a one-time visit to the clinic; they demand consistent care, daily habits, and a lifestyle that supports skin health from the inside out.

Just as going to the gym doesn't replace a healthy diet and lifestyle, cosmetic treatments must be supported by long-term maintenance to ensure results not only last but also evolve gracefully with you. Your skin is dynamic: affected by age, hormones, environment, and stress. Without ongoing care, even the best treatments will eventually fade. But when you take a proactive approach, combining professional treatments with personalised home care, sun protection, and lifestyle choices, you empower your skin to thrive for years to come.

11

Maintaining Results & Healthy Skin Habits

POST-TREATMENT CARE ESSENTIALS

The first few days following any cosmetic treatment are crucial. This is when your skin is at its most vulnerable and needs support to heal, repair, and integrate the changes from your procedure.

Following your practitioner's aftercare instructions exactly is essential. These guidelines are based on clinical evidence and designed to minimise the risk of infection, inflammation, or suboptimal results. Skipping steps or applying products too soon can interfere with healing or trigger unnecessary irritation. Most treatments come with short-term side effects, including mild swelling, redness, or tightness. These symptoms are typical and typically resolve within hours or days but knowing what's expected vs. what's not is essential.

Be especially mindful in the first 24 to 72 hours. Avoid applying makeup unless advised, and hold off on active ingredients like retinol, exfoliating acids, or vitamin C serums. Skip saunas, intense workouts, or anything that raises the skin's temperature, as this can increase swelling or delay recovery. If something feels off, such as increasing pain, pus, or prolonged swelling, don't wait to ask questions. Your practitioner is there to support you beyond the treatment room.

REGULAR PROFESSIONAL TREATMENTS

Cosmetic treatments work best when they're seen as part of a larger rhythm of care. Just like dental check-ups or haircuts, your skin needs regular professional attention to stay at its healthiest. One session may bring a beautiful boost, but it's the follow-up care that maintains and enhances your results over time.

Different skin treatments are often scheduled at varying intervals, and this can depend on factors such as the type of treatment, the specific skin concern, and individual goals. For example, some people may undergo treatments like skin needling more frequently when actively addressing issues such as pigmentation or scarring, before moving to less frequent sessions for ongoing maintenance. Light-based or energy-based therapies, such as IPL or fractional laser, may also be spaced out over the year depending on the technology used and practitioner guidance. Because every skin type and concern is unique, it's important to discuss timing and frequency with a qualified health professional who can provide recommendations tailored to your needs.

Your treatment plan should be individualised and flexible. As your skin changes with age, hormones, or lifestyle shifts, your plan should evolve too. Regular check-ins with your practitioner allow them to assess how your skin is responding, tweak your plan, and layer treatments in a safe, complementary way. Combining clinic-based treatments with a consistent home routine significantly amplifies results and reduces the need for more aggressive interventions down the line.

DAILY SKINCARE ROUTINE

The foundation of beautiful, long-lasting skin lies in your daily routine. While professional treatments create change, it's what you do every morning and night that protects and preserves those results. A well-built skincare routine doesn't have to be complicated; it just needs to be consistent, evidence-based, and tailored to your individual needs.

Cleansing your skin gently but thoroughly helps remove makeup, pollution, sweat, and bacteria that can clog pores and dull your complexion. Following with a moisturiser appropriate for your skin type helps support the barrier and retain hydration. A healthy barrier is your skin's first line of defence, and it's often compromised post-treatment, so this step matters more than you might think.

Sun protection is the most critical step in any routine. Daily application of broad-spectrum SPF 50 helps protect against UV rays that cause over 80% of visible aging. Even if you're mostly indoors, incidental sun exposure through windows and screens adds up over time.

Depending on your skin goals, active ingredients can offer powerful support. Vitamin C brightens the skin and protects against environmental damage. Retinoids boost cell turnover, stimulate collagen, and smooth texture, though they should be introduced slowly and paused after specific treatments. Peptides and niacinamide offer gentle yet effective support for strengthening, calming, and renewing the skin.

The key is to build a sustainable ritual that you can maintain and enjoy, rather than chasing trends or overwhelming your skin with products. Your skin responds best to consistency, not intensity.

SUN PROTECTION

Sun exposure is the number one cause of premature aging, pigmentation, and loss of elasticity, and it's also one of the most preventable. UV radiation accelerates the breakdown of collagen, damages the skin's DNA, and increases inflammation. After any cosmetic procedure, your skin is often more sensitive to light, making sun protection even more essential to preserve your results and prevent post-inflammatory pigmentation.

Daily use of a broad-spectrum sunscreen with SPF 50 is non-negotiable. Choose a product that offers protection from both UVA (aging) and UVB (burning) rays. Apply generously every morning and reapply throughout the day, especially if you're outdoors or sweating.

In addition to sunscreen, physical protection is highly effective. Wide-brim hats, sunglasses, and UPF-rated clothing can shield the face and neck from incidental exposure. When possible, avoid direct sunlight between 10 am and 3 pm, when UV rays are at their peak.

Post-treatment, you may need to avoid sun exposure entirely for several days to prevent irritation or pigmentation. Speak with your practitioner about your individual sun protection plan, especially after laser, micro needling, or chemical peels.

Sun protection isn't just about damage prevention; it's the cornerstone of healthy aging and treatment longevity.

HEALTHY LIFESTYLE HABITS FOR SKIN

Your skin is your body's largest organ, and it reflects the quality of your internal health. No treatment or skincare routine can fully compensate for chronic stress, poor diet, or lack of sleep. That's why one of the most impactful ways to maintain your skin results is to live a skin-supportive lifestyle.

A balanced diet fuels your skin with the nutrients it needs to repair, renew, and defend itself. Antioxidant-rich foods like berries, leafy greens, nuts, and seeds help fight oxidative stress. Omega-3 fatty acids found in salmon, flaxseed, and walnuts reduce inflammation and support a healthy skin barrier. Protein, the building block of collagen, is also essential for repair and structure.

Sleep is when your skin regenerates. During deep sleep, the body releases growth hormone, repairs cellular damage, and produces collagen. Aim for 7 to 9 hours of quality sleep each night and try to keep your routine consistent even on weekends.

Managing stress is equally important. Chronic stress elevates cortisol levels, which break down collagen and trigger inflammation. Simple rituals like journaling, movement, deep breathing, or unplugging from screens can reduce stress and improve skin health from within.

Smoking and excessive alcohol not only deplete nutrients but also speed up aging. Both restrict blood flow to the skin, decrease oxygen delivery, and impair collagen production. Avoiding or minimising these habits can dramatically extend the life of your treatments and your skin.

HYDRATION AND SKIN HEALTH

Hydration is often underestimated in skincare, but it plays a critical role in how your skin looks, feels, and functions. Dehydrated skin can appear dull, crepey, or inflamed, and it's more prone to fine lines, flaking, and irritation, especially after cosmetic treatments.

Start with internal hydration. Most people need around 2 to 3 litres of water per day, depending on climate, activity levels, and health status. Consuming water-rich foods like cucumbers, watermelon, and leafy greens also supports cellular hydration.

Typically, hydrating skincare can make a dramatic difference. Humectants like hyaluronic acid and glycerin draw water into the skin. Occlusives like squalane, ceramides, or balms help trap that hydration in place, preventing moisture loss. Hydrating masks and mists can be used weekly or as needed to boost comfort and glow.

After treatments like laser or micro needling, the skin may lose moisture more easily, so prioritising hydration helps support healing and prevents barrier disruption. Hydrated skin is also more receptive to active ingredients and more resilient against environmental stress.

AVOIDING HARMFUL BEHAVIOURS

While there are many things you can do to support your skin, there are also a few habits to avoid if you want to protect your investment. Some of the most common skincare mistakes are subtle but can sabotage your results.

Picking or squeezing blemishes may be tempting, but it increases inflammation, causes scarring, and spreads bacteria. If you're dealing with persistent congestion or breakouts, seek professional extractions or targeted treatments.

Over-exfoliating is another common issue. While exfoliation has its place, too much can strip the skin barrier, cause micro-tears, and lead to chronic redness or flakiness. Limit exfoliation to one or two times a week and avoid using multiple exfoliants at once.

Ignoring your skin's signals can also be problematic. If you notice irritation, sudden breakouts, or unusual pigmentation, don't delay follow-up or self-diagnose with new products. Consult your practitioner to rule out reactions and get personalised advice.

Finally, don't rush back into active products or harsh treatments after a procedure. Let your skin heal before reintroducing ingredients like retinol or acids. Respect your skin's natural pace.

MONITORING YOUR SKIN OVER TIME

Just like our bodies and minds, our skin evolves. What worked in your 20s might not work in your 40s, and your treatment needs will shift with age, environment, hormones, and health. Learning to observe your skin with curiosity and care is one of the best things you can do for long-term confidence.

Regular self-checks allow you to track texture changes, pigmentation, or new concerns. Monthly or seasonal observations, especially when tied to your menstrual cycle, stress levels, or diet. As this can help you notice patterns and pre-empt flare-ups. Consider keeping a skin journal or photo log to track changes over time.

Check in with your practitioner every few months, or whenever your skin feels different. These visits aren't just for treatments; they're opportunities to reassess your plan, explore new options, and stay proactive in your skin journey.

As you age, your skin goals may shift, too. You might begin focusing more on texture, hydration, or lifting. Staying in tune with your skin's evolution allows you to age with intention rather than resistance.

EMPOWERING YOU FOR LONG-TERM SKIN CONFIDENCE

At the heart of it all, skincare isn't about perfection; it's about confidence, consistency, and connection. When you understand your skin, treat it kindly, and support it through thoughtful habits and professional care, you build more than just a skincare routine; you build trust with yourself.

Long-term skin confidence comes from setting realistic expectations, committing to maintenance, and understanding that aging is not a problem to be solved, but a process to be supported. The more sustainable your approach, the more effortless your results become.

Work with your practitioner as a collaborative partner in your journey. Ask questions, share concerns, and revisit your goals regularly. Together, you can adapt your plan as your skin and life evolve.

Remember, your glow doesn't come from a single product or appointment. It comes from the small, consistent choices you make every day. And when you care for your skin with love, patience, and purpose, that glow becomes something no treatment can replicate; it's yours.

Disclaimer

This book is intended for educational and informational purposes only and is not a substitute for professional medical advice, diagnosis, or treatment. The content reflects the professional knowledge, training, and clinical experience of the author, a registered cosmetic nurse. It is designed to help readers better understand skin health and non-surgical cosmetic treatments.

All medical procedures, including injectable and laser treatments, carry risks and potential complications. Individual outcomes vary and are influenced by a range of factors, including skin type, health status, and practitioner technique. No guarantees of results are made or implied.

Readers are encouraged to seek personalised advice and assessment from a qualified healthcare professional before undergoing any cosmetic procedure. The author does not endorse or recommend any specific product, device, or brand unless clearly stated as part of an educational example.

This publication complies with the AHPRA Guidelines for Advertising a Regulated Health Service. It does not include testimonials or before-and-after photographs, and all efforts have been made to ensure the information is accurate, evidence-based, and in line with current professional standards at the time of publication.

Reference list

Baldwin, H. and Tan, J. (2020). Effects of Diet on Acne and Its Response to Treatment. *American Journal of Clinical Dermatology*, [online] 22(1). doi: https://doi.org/10.1007/s40257-020-00542-y.

Brenner, M. and Hearing, V.J. (2007). The protective role of melanin against UV damage in human skin. *Photochemistry and Photobiology*, [online] 84(3), pp.539–549. Doi: HTTPs://doi.org/10.1111/j.1751-1097.2007.00226.x.

Dhabale, A. and Nagpure, S. (2022). Types of Psoriasis and Their Effects on the Immune System. *Cureus*, [online] 14(9), p.e29536. Doi: https://doi.org/10.7759/cureus.29536.

Dréno, B. (2017). What is new in the pathophysiology of acne: an overview. *Journal of the European Academy of Dermatology and Venereology*, 31(S5), pp.8–12. doi: https://doi.org/10.1111/jdv.14374.

Falinski, J. (2024). *Fitzpatrick Scale and Skin Types.* [online] Clinilabs | The CRO for CNS. Available at: https://clinilabs.com/volunteers/fp/.

Grice, E.A. and Segre, J.A. (2011). The skin microbiome. *Nature Reviews Microbiology*, [online] 9(4), pp.244–253. doi: https://doi.org/10.1038/nrmicro2537.

Gupta, A. and Chaudhry, M. (2005). Rosacea and its management: an overview. *Journal of the European Academy of Dermatology and Venereology*, 19(3), pp.273–285. doi: https://doi.org/10.1111/j.1468-3083.2005.01216.x.

Kurokawa, I., Danby, F.W., Ju, Q., Wang, X., Xiang, L.F., Xia, L., Chen, W., Nagy, I., Picardo, M., Suh, D.H., Ganceviciene, R., Schagen, S., Tsatsou, F. and Zouboulis, C.C. (2009). New developments in our understanding of acne pathogenesis and treatment. *Experimental Dermatology*, 18(10), pp.821–832. doi: https://doi.org/10.1111/j.1600-0625.2009.00890.x.

Lakhan, M.K. and Lynch, M. (2021). Skin pigmentation. *Medicine*. Doi: https://doi.org/10.1016/j.mpmed.2021.04.010.

Raharja, A., Mahil, S.K. and Barker, J.N. (2021). Psoriasis: a brief overview. *Clinical Medicine (London, England)*, 21(3), pp.170–173. doi: https://doi.org/10.7861/clinmed.2021-0257.

Suh, D.H. and Kwon, H.H. (2015). What's new in the physiopathology of acne? *British Journal of Dermatology*, [online] 172, pp.13–19. doi: https://doi.org/10.1111/bjd.13634.

Thawabteh, A.M., Jibreen, A., Karaman, D., Thawabteh, A. and Karaman, R. (2023). Skin Pigmentation Types, Causes and Treatment—A Review. *Molecules*, [online] 28(12), p.4839. doi: https://doi.org/10.3390/molecules28124839.